PRESCRIPTION
AND
OVER-THE-COUNTER
DRUGS

GENERAL EDITORS

Dale C. Garell, M.D.

Medical Director, California Children Services, Department of Health
   Services, County of Los Angeles
Clinical Professor, Department of Pediatrics & Family Medicine,
   University of Southern California School of Medicine
Former president, Society for Adolescent Medicine

Solomon H. Snyder, M.D.

Distinguished Service Professor of Neuroscience, Pharmacology, and
   Psychiatry, Johns Hopkins University School of Medicine
Former president, Society of Neuroscience
Albert Lasker Award in Medical Research, 1978

CONSULTING EDITORS

Robert W. Blum, M.D., Ph.D.

Associate Professor, School of Public Health and Department of
   Pediatrics
Director, Adolescent Health Program, University of Minnesota
Consultant, World Health Organization

Charles E. Irwin, Jr., M.D.

Associate Professor of Pediatrics
Director, Division of Adolescent Medicine,
   University of California, San Francisco

Lloyd J. Kolbe, Ph.D.

Chief, Office of School Health & Special Projects, Center for Health
   Promotion & Education, Centers for Disease Control
President, American School Health Association

Jordan J. Popkin

Director, Division of Federal Employee Occupational Health, U.S. Public
   Health Service Region I

Joseph L. Rauh, M.D.

Professor of Pediatrics and Medicine, Adolescent Medicine, Children's
   Hospital Medical Center, Cincinnati
Former president, Society for Adolescent Medicine

THE ENCYCLOPEDIA OF
H E A L T H

MEDICAL DISORDERS
AND THEIR TREATMENT

Dale C. Garell, M.D. · General Editor

PRESCRIPTION AND OVER-THE-COUNTER DRUGS

Mary Kittredge

Introduction by C. Everett Koop, M.D., Sc.D.
Surgeon General, U.S. Public Health Service

CHELSEA HOUSE PUBLISHERS
New York · Philadelphia

The goal of the ENCYCLOPEDIA OF HEALTH *is to provide general information in the ever-changing areas of physiology, psychology, and related medical issues. The titles in this series are not intended to take the place of the professional advice of a physician or other health-care professional.*

Chelsea House Publishers
EDITOR-IN-CHIEF Nancy Toff
EXECUTIVE EDITOR Remmel T. Nunn
MANAGING EDITOR Karyn Gullen Browne
COPY CHIEF Juliann Barbato
PICTURE EDITOR Adrian G. Allen
ART DIRECTOR Maria Epes
MANUFACTURING MANAGER Gerald Levine

The Encyclopedia of Health
SENIOR EDITOR Sam Tanenhaus

Staff for PRESCRIPTION AND OVER-THE-COUNTER DRUGS
COPY EDITOR Lisa Fenev
DEPUTY COPY CHIEF Ellen Scordato
EDITORIAL ASSISTANT Jennifer Trachtenberg
PICTURE RESEARCHER Nisa Rauschenberg
ASSISTANT ART DIRECTOR Lorraine Machlin
SENIOR DESIGNER Marjorie Zaum
PRODUCTION COORDINATOR Joseph Romano

First Printing

1 3 5 7 9 8 6 4 2

Library of Congress Cataloging-in-Publication Data

Kittredge, Mary, 1949–
  PRESCRIPTION AND OVER-THE-COUNTER DRUGS / Mary Kittredge; introduction by C. Everett Koop.
    p. cm. — (The Encyclopedia of health. Medical disorders and their treatment)
  Bibliography: p.
  Includes index.
  Summary: Discusses the world of prescription and nonprescription drugs, exploring such aspects as generic drugs and those obtained with a doctor's order.
  ISBN 0-7910-0062-1.
      0-7910-0502-X (pbk.)
  1. Drugs—Juvenile literature. 2. Drugs, Nonprescription—Juvenile literature. [1. Drugs. 2. Drugs, Nonprescription.]
  I. Title. II. Series.   88-34173
RM301.17.K58 1989   CIP
615'.1—dc19   AC

CONTENTS

THE ENCYCLOPEDIA OF
H E A L T H

THE HEALTHY BODY

The Circulatory System
Dental Health
The Digestive System
The Endocrine System
Exercise
Genetics & Heredity
The Human Body: An Overview
Hygiene
The Immune System
Memory & Learning
The Musculoskeletal System
The Neurological System
Nutrition
The Reproductive System
The Respiratory System
The Senses
Speech & Hearing
Sports Medicine
Vision
Vitamins & Minerals

THE LIFE CYCLE

Adolescence
Adulthood
Aging
Childhood
Death & Dying
The Family
Friendship & Love
Pregnancy & Birth

MEDICAL ISSUES

Careers in Health Care
Environmental Health
Folk Medicine
Health Care Delivery
Holistic Medicine
Medical Ethics
Medical Fakes & Frauds
Medical Technology
Medicine & the Law
Occupational Health
Public Health

PSYCHOLOGICAL DISORDERS AND THEIR TREATMENT

Anxiety & Phobias
Child Abuse
Compulsive Behavior
Delinquency & Criminal Behavior
Depression
Diagnosing & Treating Mental Illness
Eating Habits & Disorders
Learning Disabilities
Mental Retardation
Personality Disorders
Schizophrenia
Stress Management
Suicide

MEDICAL DISORDERS AND THEIR TREATMENT

AIDS
Allergies
Alzheimer's Disease
Arthritis
Birth Defects
Cancer
The Common Cold
Diabetes
First Aid & Emergency Medicine
Gynecological Disorders
Headaches
The Hospital
Kidney Disorders
Medical Diagnosis
The Mind-Body Connection
Mononucleosis and Other Infectious Diseases
Nuclear Medicine
Organ Transplants
Pain
Physical Handicaps
Poisons & Toxins
Prescription & OTC Drugs
Sexually Transmitted Diseases
Skin Disorders
Stroke & Heart Disease
Substance Abuse
Tropical Medicine

PREVENTION AND EDUCATION: THE KEYS TO GOOD HEALTH

C. Everett Koop, M.D., Sc.D.
Surgeon General,
U.S. Public Health Service

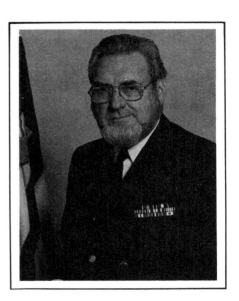

The issue of health education has received particular attention in recent years because of the presence of AIDS in the news. But our response to this particular tragedy points up a number of broader issues that doctors, public health officials, educators, and the public face. In particular, it points up the necessity for sound health education for citizens of all ages.

Over the past 25 years this country has been able to bring about dramatic declines in the death rates for heart disease, stroke, accidents, and, for people under the age of 45, cancer. Today, Americans generally eat better and take better care of themselves than ever before. Thus, with the help of modern science and technology, they have a better chance of surviving serious—even catastrophic— illnesses. That's the good news.

But, like every phonograph record, there's a flip side, and one with special significance for young adults. According to a report issued in 1979 by Dr. Julius Richmond, my predecessor as Surgeon General, Americans aged 15 to 24 had a higher death rate in 1979 than they did 20 years earlier. The causes: violent death and injury, alcohol and drug abuse, unwanted pregnancies, and sexually transmitted diseases. Adolescents are particularly vulnerable, because they are beginning to explore their own sexuality and perhaps to experiment with drugs. The need for educating young people is critical, and the price of neglect is high.

Yet even for the population as a whole, our health is still far from what it could be. Why? A 1974 Canadian government report attributed all death and disease to four broad elements: inadequacies in the health-care system, behavioral factors or unhealthy life-styles, environmental hazards, and human biological factors.

To be sure, there are diseases that are still beyond the control of even our advanced medical knowledge and techniques. And despite yearnings that are as old as the human race itself, there is no "fountain of youth" to ward off aging and death. Still, there is a solution to many of the problems that undermine sound health. In a word, that solution is prevention. Prevention, which includes health promotion and education, saves lives, improves the quality of life, and, in the long run, saves money.

In the United States, organized public health activities and preventive medicine have a long history. Important milestones include the improvement of sanitary procedures and the development of pasteurized milk in the late 19th century, and the introduction in the mid-20th century of effective vaccines against polio, measles, German measles, mumps, and other once-rampant diseases. Internationally, organized public health efforts began on a wide-scale basis with the International Sanitary Conference of 1851, to which 12 nations sent representatives. The World Health Organization, founded in 1948, continues these efforts under the aegis of the United Nations, with particular emphasis on combatting communicable diseases and the training of health-care workers.

But despite these accomplishments, much remains to be done in the field of prevention. For too long, we have had a medical care system that is science- and technology-based, focused, essentially, on illness and mortality. It is now patently obvious that both the social and the economic costs of such a system are becoming insupportable.

Implementing prevention—and its corollaries, health education and promotion—is the job of several groups of people:

First, the medical and scientific professions need to continue basic scientific research, and here we are making considerable progress. But increased concern with prevention will also have a decided impact on how primary-care doctors practice medicine. With a shift to health-based rather than morbidity-based medicine, the role of the "new physician" will include a healthy dose of patient education.

Second, practitioners of the social and behavioral sciences—psychologists, economists, city planners—along with lawyers, business leaders, and government officials—must solve the practical and ethical dilemmas confronting us: poverty, crime, civil rights, literacy, education, employment, housing, sanitation, environmental protection, health care delivery systems, and so forth. All of these issues affect public health.

Third is the public at large. We'll consider that very important group in a moment.

Fourth, and the linchpin in this effort, is the public health profession—doctors, epidemiologists, teachers—who must harness the professional expertise of the first two groups and the common sense and cooperation of the third, the public. They must define the problems statistically and qualitatively and then help us set priorities for finding the solutions.

To a very large extent, improving those statistics is the responsibility of every individual. So let's consider more specifically what the role of the individual should be and why health education is so important to that role. First, and most obviously, individuals can protect themselves from illness and injury and thus minimize their need for professional medical care. They can eat a nutritious diet, get adequate exercise, avoid tobacco, alcohol, and drugs, and take prudent steps to avoid accidents. The proverbial "apple a day keeps the doctor away" is not so far from the truth, after all.

Second, individuals should actively participate in their own medical care. They should schedule regular medical and dental checkups. Should they develop an illness or injury, they should know when to treat themselves and when to seek professional help. To gain the maximum benefit from any medical treatment that they do require, individuals must become partners in that treatment. For instance, they should understand the effects and side effects of medications. I counsel young physicians that there is no such thing as too much information when talking with patients. But the corollary is the patient must know enough about the nuts and bolts of the healing process to understand what the doctor is telling him. That is at least partially the patient's responsibility.

Education is equally necessary for us to understand the ethical and public policy issues in health care today. Sometimes individuals will encounter these issues in making decisions about their own treatment or that of family members. Other citizens may encounter them as jurors in medical malpractice cases. But we all become involved, indirectly, when we elect our public officials, from school board members to the president. Should surrogate parenting be legal? To what extent is drug testing desirable, legal, or necessary? Should there be public funding for family planning, hospitals, various types of medical research, and medical care for the indigent? How should we allocate scant technological resources, such as kidney dialysis and organ transplants? What is the proper role of government in protecting the rights of patients?

What are the broad goals of public health in the United States today? In 1980, the Public Health Service issued a report aptly entitled *Promoting Health-Preventing Disease: Objectives for the Nation.* This report expressed its goals in terms of mortality and in terms of intermediate goals in education and health improvement. It identified 15 major concerns: controlling high blood pressure; improving family planning; improving pregnancy care and infant health; increasing the rate of immunization; controlling sexually transmitted diseases; controlling the presence of toxic agents and radiation in the environment; improving occupational safety and health; preventing accidents; promoting water fluoridation and dental health; controlling infectious diseases; decreasing smoking; decreasing alcohol and drug abuse; improving nutrition; promoting physical fitness and exercise; and controlling stress and violent behavior.

For healthy adolescents and young adults (ages 15 to 24), the specific goal was a 20% reduction in deaths, with a special focus on motor vehicle injuries and alcohol and drug abuse. For adults (ages 25 to 64), the aim was 25% fewer deaths, with a concentration on heart attacks, strokes, and cancers.

Smoking is perhaps the best example of how individual behavior can have a direct impact on health. Today cigarette smoking is recognized as the most important single preventable cause of death in our society. It is responsible for more cancers and more cancer deaths than any other known agent; is a prime risk factor for heart and blood vessel disease, chronic bronchitis, and emphysema; and is a frequent cause of complications in pregnancies and of babies born prematurely, underweight, or with potentially fatal respiratory and cardiovascular problems.

Since the release of the Surgeon General's first report on smoking in 1964, the proportion of adult smokers has declined substantially, from 43% in 1965 to 30.5% in 1985. Since 1965, 37 million people have quit smoking. Although there is still much work to be done if we are to become a "smoke-free society," it is heartening to note that public health and public education efforts—such as warnings on cigarette packages and bans on broadcast advertising—have already had significant effects.

In 1835, Alexis de Tocqueville, a French visitor to America, wrote, "In America the passion for physical well-being is general." Today, as then, health and fitness are front-page items. But with the greater scientific and technological resources now available to us, we are in a far stronger position to make good health care available to everyone. And with the greater technological threats to us as we approach the 21st century, the need to do so is more urgent than ever before. Comprehensive information about basic biology, preventive medicine, medical and surgical treatments, and related ethical and public policy issues can help you arm yourself with the knowledge you need to be healthy throughout your life.

FOREWORD

Dale C. Garell, M.D.

Advances in our understanding of health and disease during the 20th century have been truly remarkable. Indeed, it could be argued that modern health care is one of the greatest accomplishments in all of human history. In the early 1900s, improvements in sanitation, water treatment, and sewage disposal reduced death rates and increased longevity. Previously untreatable illnesses can now be managed with antibiotics, immunizations, and modern surgical techniques. Discoveries in the fields of immunology, genetic diagnosis, and organ transplantation are revolutionizing the prevention and treatment of disease. Modern medicine is even making inroads against cancer and heart disease, two of the leading causes of death in the United States.

Although there is much to be proud of, medicine continues to face enormous challenges. Science has vanquished diseases such as smallpox and polio, but new killers, most notably AIDS, confront us. Moreover, we now victimize ourselves with what some have called "diseases of choice," or those brought on by drug and alcohol abuse, bad eating habits, and mismanagement of the stresses and strains of contemporary life. The very technology that is doing so much to prolong life has brought with it previously unimaginable ethical dilemmas related to issues of death and dying. The rising cost of health-care is a matter of central concern to us all. And violence in the form of automobile accidents, homicide, and suicide remain the major killers of young adults.

In the past, most people were content to leave health care and medical treatment in the hands of professionals. But since the 1960s, the consumer of medical care—that is, the patient—has assumed an increasingly central role in the management of his or her own health. There has also been a new emphasis placed on prevention: People are recognizing that their own actions can help prevent many of the conditions that have caused death and disease in the past. This accounts for the growing commitment to good nutrition and regular exercise, for the fact that more and more people are choosing not to smoke, and for a new moderation in people's drinking habits.

People want to know more about themselves and their own health. They are curious about their body: its anatomy, physiology, and biochemistry. They want to keep up with rapidly evolving medical technologies and procedures. They are willing to educate themselves about common disorders and diseases so that they can be full partners in their own health-care.

The ENCYCLOPEDIA OF HEALTH is designed to provide the basic knowledge that readers will need if they are to take significant responsibility for their own health. It is also meant to serve as a frame of reference for further study and exploration. The ENCYCLOPEDIA is divided into five subsections: The Healthy Body; The Life Cycle; Medical Disorders & Their Treatment; Psychological Disorders & Their Treatment; and Medical Issues. For each topic covered by the ENCYCLOPEDIA, we present the essential facts about the relevant biology; the symptoms, diagnosis, and treatment of common diseases and disorders; and ways in which you can prevent or reduce the severity of health problems when that is possible. The ENCYCLOPEDIA also projects what may lie ahead in the way of future treatment or prevention strategies.

The broad range of topics and issues covered in the ENCYCLOPEDIA reflects the fact that human health encompasses physical, psychological, social, environmental, and spiritual well-being. Just as the mind and the body are inextricably linked, so, too, is the individual an integral part of the wider world that comprises his or her family, society, and environment. To discuss health in its broadest aspect it is necessary to explore the many ways in which it is connected to such fields as law, social science, public policy, economics, and even religion. And so, the ENCYCLOPEDIA is meant to be a bridge between science, medical technology, the world at large, and you. I hope that it will inspire you to pursue in greater depth particular areas of interest, and that you will take advantage of the suggestions for further reading and the lists of resources and organizations that can provide additional information.

THE WORLD OF DRUGS

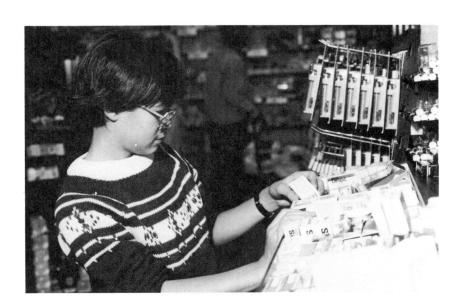

In the early 1900s, when physician Sir William Osler wrote, "Nothing so distinguishes man from the animals as the desire to take medicine," he hit the mark not just for his era but also for our own. For, as medical science finds new medicines for major diseases and as ads promote new over-the-counter (OTC) remedies for minor ills, Americans buy more drugs of all sorts than ever before. Nonprescription pain relievers alone account for $700 million of the more than $3 billion spent each year on OTC drugs, and each year doctors write 1.5 billion orders for "prescription only" drugs that cost consumers a total of more than $26 billion.

Who takes all these drugs? Almost everyone, young and old alike. Indeed, a recent survey commissioned by Bristol-Meyers, a leading drug manufacturer, reported that young people suffer many of the minor ailments for which adults take medicines: Seventy-three percent of the young-adult population suffers at least one headache a year; 56% get backaches; and more than 40% get stomach pains. Young people are also stricken by illnesses that are comparatively rare among adults, including chicken pox (a childhood disease) and mononucleosis (common among young adults); pain caused by developing wisdom teeth; skin eruptions; and sports injuries.

Like adults, young people view drugs ambivalently. They sometimes have trouble distinguishing useful remedies from useless ones and can fall prey to advertising claims for OTC drugs that promise miraculous cures, especially for cosmetic problems such as acne. At the same time, young people also tend to equate all drugs, even those prescribed by physicians, with illegal substances; many worry they will become dependent on them. Thus, they may refuse drugs that are vital to their health.

It is difficult to make wise choices about drugs—OTC or prescribed—when good information is scarce or confusing, when the media daily push new remedies at us, and when even useful drugs can have distressing side effects. This book describes both the advances and dangers of modern medicine. The following chapters explain the facts about prescription and OTC drugs: what they are; how they work; what their side effects may be; how to buy and take OTC and prescribed drugs safely; how scientists and businesses develop and market new drugs; how government agencies help regulate them; what ingredients are contained in some common OTC and prescribed drugs; how victims of extremely rare ailments benefit from new drugs; where the next "miracle drugs" may come from and what they may be; and how to get more thorough information about prescription and OTC drugs.

•   •   •   •

CHAPTER 1

. . . .

FROM THE PRIMITIVE TO THE PRESENT

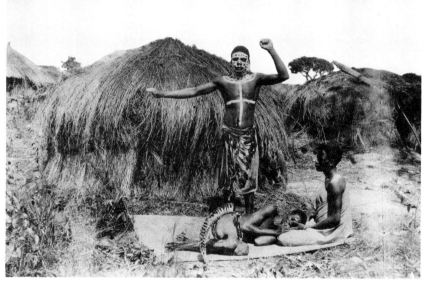

Nigerian medicine man.

The first efforts made by humans to keep or regain their health stemmed from their ideas of how sickness began. Neanderthals, who seem to have thought evil spirits caused disease, devised cures that involved magic rituals and employed magic substances found in minerals, plants, and animal parts. More advanced remedies developed about 10,000 years ago, during the new Stone Age. The people who lived in this era built huts, polished stone tools, raised animals and plants for food, and performed trephination, a kind of skull surgery still practiced today. Ancient surgeons thought the operation released demons causing pain inside the head; modern surgeons realize the operation can relieve pressure built up by excess bleeding inside the skull. It is also likely that inhabitants of the Stone Age developed herbal cures.

ANCIENT MEDICINES

Our first certain knowledge of ancient medicines comes from the Egyptians. Beginning in about 3,500 B.C., Egyptian healers composed instructions for diagnosing and treating diseases and recorded them on papyrus, paper made from reeds.

Like the cures of earlier peoples, Egyptian remedies reflected their religious beliefs. Two Egyptian gods associated with medicine were Thoth, the patron of physicians, and Horus, the protector of humans against dangerous animals. Healers called upon these divine figures to drive evil spirits out of a sufferer, and they administered drugs—"hateful remedies"—as part of the ritual.

Egyptian physicians tested hundreds of drugs: metals, such as copper and antimony; foods, such as figs, beans, and onions; alcoholic beverages, such as beer and wine; and parts of animals, such as ox liver and brains. Healers tried different remedies until they found one that cured a specific ailment. This experimental practice, which remains the basis of modern drug therapy, yielded many effective cures. Copper, alum, and aluminous clay, which the Egyptians used to combat trachoma (a parasitic infection of the eye), are recognized as useful ingredients by con-

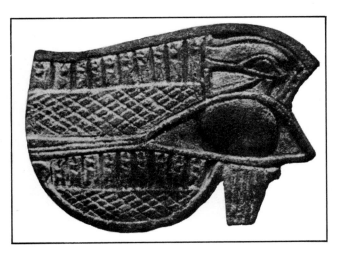

Healers in ancient Egypt relied on superstition as well as on experimentation. This amulet, or charm, is inscribed with the eye of Horus, the god said to ward off attacks from dangerous beasts.

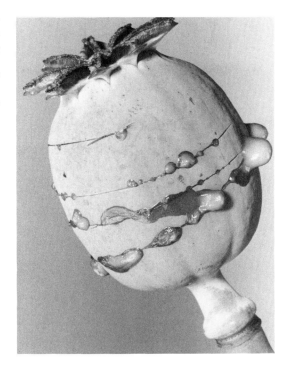

Mesopotamian healers derived medications from 250 different herbs, including Papaver sominiferum *(the poppy plant), which, when slit, drips raw opium, a powerful narcotic.*

temporary physicians. So is the use of moldy bread—which foreshadowed antibiotics—for treating infections, as well as yeast, which presaged our use of vitamins. Other Egyptian potions proved less enduring, such as concoctions made of fly dirt, pelican droppings, human urine, gazelle dung, and crocodile dung. Such cures, and others equally repellent, most likely sprang from the element of Egyptian medical theory that held, "if the demon [is] disgusted, it will leave" the body.

At about the same time, the Mesopotamians, who dwelled in the fertile land between the Tigris and Euphrates rivers, also wrote down medical treatments that depended as much on religion as they did on drugs. Mesopotamian healers fell into three groups: diviners, who interpreted omens; priests, whose prayers expelled evil spirits; and physicians, who performed surgery and administered remedies. These remedies were drawn from about 120 minerals and 250 different herbs, including the poppy (the source of opium), and belladonna, which remains a useful ingredient in medications prescribed for spasms, coughing, and asthma.

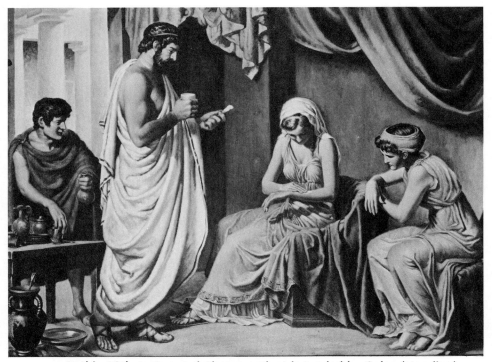

In this 19th-century painting, a patient is tended by Galen (standing), the ancient Greek physician whose systematic compilation of medical knowledge remained the foundation of Western medical practice for 1,500 years.

By about 600 B.C., medicine began to be practiced in a scientific way—in Greece, where physicians developed a truly systematic approach to healing. For instance, they adjusted existing treatments on the basis of their careful observation of patients. Drugs ranked low among treatments recommended by the physician Hippocrates, "the Father of Modern Medicine," who favored rest and changes in diet.

The greatest doctor in ancient Rome was probably Galen (A.D. 129–99), who collected the medical knowledge of antiquity, combined it with his own vast knowledge, and created a system that remained the foundation of medical practice in the West for 1,500 years. Roman physicians commonly prescribed drugs along with rest, fresh air, and mineral baths. Many, however, continued to rely on prayer; the Romans believed disease was a form of punishment sent by angry gods, and that appeasing them was the best cure.

Eastern cultures also developed sophisticated remedies. At

least as early as 500 B.C.—and probably long before—healers in India used more than 500 different drugs, including rauwolfia, a sedative that also lowered blood pressure; kushta, a plant that helped people with eye trouble; and soma, a painkilling herb so potent it bore the name of an Indian god. Ancient Chinese doctors also developed effective drugs. They treated coughing with fir bark (later found to contain ephedrine, an ingredient still used in respiratory medicines) and treated leprosy by prescribing chaulmoogra oil (still the standard treatment, in purified form). Chinese physicians even vaccinated patients against smallpox centuries before the procedure occurred to European doctors.

SLOW GAINS

In the West, medical knowledge slowed after the fall of the Roman Empire in the 5th century A.D.. Indeed, from that time until A.D. 1200, medicine was practiced mostly by Christian monks who preferred to recycle remedies recommended in antiquated medical treatises rather than to devise new ones. Not until about 1500 did the spirit of experimentation awaken in Europe, when two brilliant men, Italy's Leonardo da Vinci (1452–1519) and Belgium's Andreas Vesalius (1514–64), independently studied human anatomy and thereby shed light on the structure

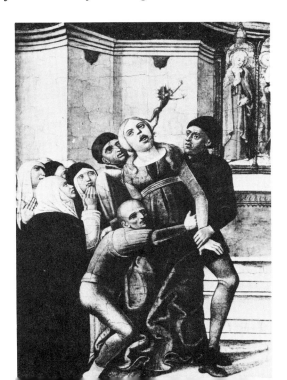

In this 15th-century painting, Saint Catherine of Siena, Italy, drives an evil spirit from the body of a patient.

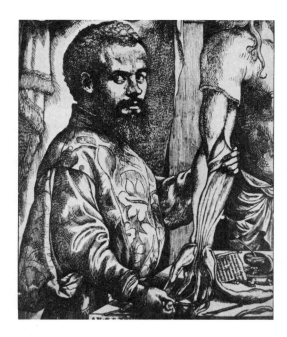

Belgian Andreas Vesalius (1514–64), a pioneer of anatomical study, made drawings that still adorn the pages of medical books.

of the body and its possible ways of malfunctioning. Important discoveries were also made in botany (the study of plant life), which brought into favor new plant-based drugs—such as quinine, ipecac, and tobacco—many of them made from plants found in North and South America by European explorers and colonists.

In the next century, scientists began to study germs and their relation to disease. In 1683, the Dutch scientist Antonie van Leeuwenhoek saw bacteria through the lens of a microscope, though concrete knowledge about germs developed slowly. Nearly 100 years passed before the English physician Sir William Jenner injected a boy with tissue from a cow that had cowpox. And even Jenner could not explain why the vaccine protected the boy from the dreaded smallpox. Jenner's method, like most medical treatment of his time, was still mostly empirical—based on trial and error. Doctors knew some drugs worked and others did not, but the reasons remained mysterious. Fields such as anatomy (the study of body structure), physiology (how the body works), pathophysiology (the effect of diseases on the body), and bacteriology (the study of germs) were not yet advanced enough to illuminate the ways in which drugs combat disease.

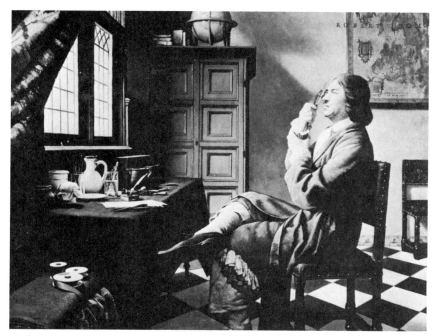

In 1683, Dutch scientist Antonie van Leeuwenhoek spied bacteria through the lens of a microscope and thus inaugurated the study of germs and their causal relation to disease.

TOWARD THE PRESENT

Great strides were made in the 19th century when French scientist Louis Pasteur (1822–95) proved that germs could cause disease and could be transmitted in some ways but not in others. His 1881 experiment, in which he weakened the germ that causes anthrax, an infectious disease, showed that the ailment could be prevented with a vaccine made not from a lesser disease, as Jenner's had been, but from anthrax itself. Meanwhile, the German scientist Robert Koch (1843–1910) developed ways of studying germs and in 1881 identified the germ responsible for tuberculosis. During the next 25 years, scientists identified more than 20 bacteria, including those that caused typhoid, botulism, diphtheria, and meningitis.

As a consequence of these discoveries, a new question arose, namely, how could these organisms be killed without harming the person infected with them? In 1928, Sir Alexander Fleming, a British doctor, observed that a mold invading one of his ex-

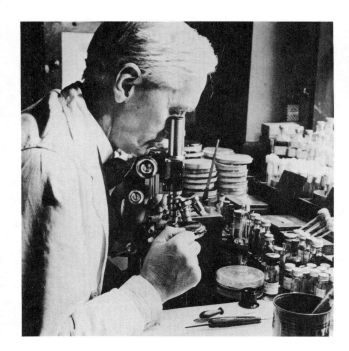

In 1928, Sir Alexander Fleming stumbled onto penicillin when a mold killed the bacteria he had been trying to grow in one of his experiments.

periments killed the bacteria he had been trying to grow. The mold was *Penicillium notatum*—the first penicillin. It was first tried on humans in 1941 and paved the way for further development of antibiotics such as actinomycin, Aureomycin, streptinomycin, chloramphenicol, and others.

Parallel advances in research helped counteract another major medical problem: pain. In 1806, German scientist Frederick Serteurner located morphine, an active painkilling ingredient, in the opium plant. In 1857, cocaine was isolated from the South American coca leaf. Europeans and Americans tried anesthetic gases: chloroform, nitrous oxide (laughing gas), and ether. In 1845, Horace Wells, a Connecticut dentist, had one of his own teeth pulled after he was anesthetized by nitrous oxide. The following year, London surgeon Robert Liston gave a patient ether and then amputated his leg painlessly.

Painkilling drugs not only advanced surgery and dentistry; they also formed the bases for some effective "OTC" medicines, for in those days no prescription was needed even for powerful narcotics. Thus, in the 19th century, manufacturers marketed cocaine toothache drops and morphine stomach powders, heroin headache pills, and dozens more nostrums guaranteed to "cure what ailed you."

But these remedies packed a potent, sometimes deadly punch, and hundreds of thousands of people grew addicted to them. The situation became so alarming in the United States that in 1914 the U.S. Congress passed the Harrison Act, which required licenses for doctors who prescribed narcotics and made it illegal for pharmacists to sell the drugs to patients who lacked proper prescriptions.

THE MODERN AGE

Not all drugs needed to be regulated. Aspirin, for instance, had long been known to American Indians, who introduced it to European colonists as castoreum (although the remedy also contained beaver testicles and so was thought too disgusting for common use). In the 20th century, researchers at the Bayer Company, in Germany, isolated salicylic acid from willow bark and created a synthetic substance, acetylsalicylic acid, which—under the name of aspirin and in products such as Bromo-Seltzer—

Slickly packaged cure-alls became so widespread in the United States that in 1914 Congress passed the Harrison Act, which established regulations for the prescription and sale of medications.

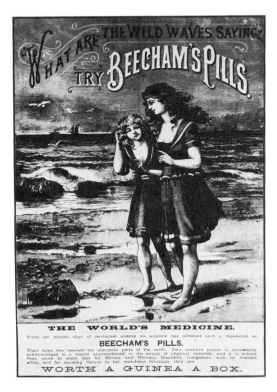

THE WORLD'S MEDICINE.

From the earliest days of medicinal science no antidote has achieved such a reputation as

BEECHAM'S PILLS.

Their fame has reached the uttermost parts of the earth; their curative power is universally acknowledged to a degree unprecedented in the annals of physical research; and it is echoed from shore to shore that for Bilious and Nervous Disorders, Indigestion with its dreaded allies, and for assisting Nature in her wondrous functions, they are

WORTH A GUINEA A BOX.

rapidly became the safest and most popular remedy that provided simple pain relief. Not until the 1980s, however, could scientists explain how it worked.

Another remedy said to have originated with American Indians was a bogus brand of cure-all manufactured in Clintonville, Connecticut, around 1900. It was sold under the name Kickapoo and hawked by a traveling band of hucksters dressed in "Indian" costumes. The Kickapoo cures included Sagwa Oil ("good for man or beast"), Indian Prairie Plant ("for female complaints"), Indian Oil, Salve, Cough Cure, Pills, and Worm Killer. All these remedies featured the same two main ingredients, molasses and rum.

Around the same time, Lydia E. Pinkham, a native of Lynn, Massachusetts, made a concoction of roots and herbs, including true unicorn (*Aletris*) and pleurisy root (*Asclepias*), that she called Lydia E. Pinkham's Vegetable Compound, a tonic said to give energy and reduce nervousness. Within a few years demand was so great that it was mass-produced by a factory that employed 450 workers. Advertisements for the product made Mrs. Pinkham one of the best-known Americans of her time.

Home remedies did not entirely dominate the drug field, however. Laboratory researchers continued to find new cures. The 19th century saw the advent of anesthetics, analgesics, and vaccines, which rank among the most important medical breakthroughs of the past, and also of antiseptics (for clean surgery and wound care); insulin (which helps fight diabetes); antihistamines (which combat allergies); and drugs that today prove effective against cancer and aid in transplant operations by preventing the body from attacking foreign cells.

In the late 20th century, drugs are valuable not only in our efforts to stave off deadly ills but also in our fight to combat headache, dandruff, poison ivy, sore throat, acne, athlete's foot, stomach upset, dry skin, and hundreds of other ailments. And like many 19th-century remedies, modern OTC drugs sometimes contain potent ingredients that, if used unwisely, can do as much harm as good. That is why knowledge about drugs is more important today than ever before.

We live in an age in which cures are not only possible but common. Modern prescription and OTC drugs can ease and even save our lives. At the same time, because disease remains a universal problem, the search for more effective drugs continues.

CHAPTER 2

. . . .

WHAT ARE DRUGS?

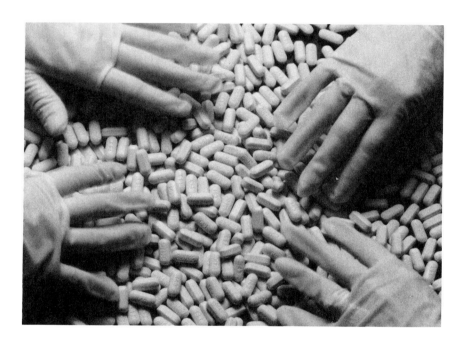

To many people, the word *drug* has come to mean an illegal substance that, when smoked, sniffed, or injected, affects the mind and body in unhealthy ways. But this definition is not entirely complete or correct, and for two reasons. First, drugs that are abused, such as cocaine and marijuana, compose just one small group of the substances people take for a vast range

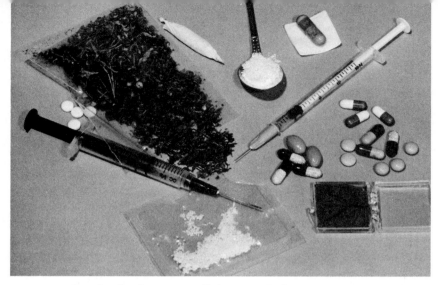

Many people mistakenly equate all drugs with illegal substances such as those shown here: marijuana, crude cocaine (in the small box), heroin (the white powder), and mood-altering pills.

of good purposes. Second, even frequently abused drugs can prove beneficial when taken under the supervision of a physician who has prescribed them for medically sound reasons.

The active ingredient in the drug marijuana, for example, the chemical tetrahydrocannabinol (THC), can ease the symptoms of glaucoma, an eye disease, and also the pain and nausea caused by cancer therapy. Cocaine, addictive and potentially lethal when abused, is prescribed by doctors to ease the pain some patients suffer from certain eye and throat surgeries. So a wider, more useful definition of the word *drug* is "a substance taken to fight ill health or to promote good health."

ORIGINS AND SOURCES

Drugs come from a huge variety of sources, from plants and animals that thrive in different parts of the globe, from creatures that dwell in the oceans, and from soil and rocks. The science of finding new drug sources in the natural world is called *pharmacognosy* (from the Greek for "recognizing drugs").

Drugs that consist of fresh or dried plant or animal material are called "crude" drugs. One such drug is ipecac, which induces vomiting and is often administered to people who have swallowed something poisonous. It consists of the dried, powdered root of the ipecacuanha plant and was used centuries ago by American Indians. Another crude drug is cod-liver oil, which is used to treat people whose diets do not contain enough vitamin A. It is obtained by boiling codfish livers in water and then skimming off the oil, which is rich in vitamin A, when it floats to the surface.

Equally simple processes can also produce mineral-based drugs. One such product is zinc, which is prescribed for people whose diets do not contain enough of the mineral or who cannot absorb it from food. Zinc is also used in a cream to protect burned flesh so it will heal faster.

Many drugs, however, cannot simply be extracted from roots, fish, or metal. Instead, they are manufactured in laboratories, where even the raw materials have been changed considerably from their most natural state. One such drug is halothane, an anesthetic gas that, when inhaled by patients prior to surgery, makes them unconscious during the operation. Halothane is produced in factories and made by mixing a gas, trichloroethylene, with the chemical hydrogen chloride. This mixture is then treated with hydrogen fluoride and bromide.

This employee of Pfizer Inc. is inspecting products for impurities, a precaution required of all American drug companies by the Food and Drug Administration (FDA).

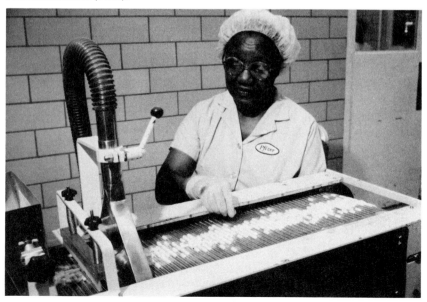

THE DRUG-BODY INTERACTION

No matter how easily a drug is made, its effect on the human body will always be complicated. This is so because drugs do not merely act on the body but interact with it. Consider how the body processes food. When eaten, food changes our bodies by building bone and tissue, giving us energy, and so on. But this process can occur only if the body, in turn, acts on the food. It must break the substance down into simple chemicals, send the chemicals to the places in the body where they are needed, and expel the waste.

So it is with drugs. Because drugs are often complex chemicals and because the body itself is complex, a book this size cannot possibly give a detailed explanation of how every drug interacts with the body. But the effect of most drugs can be described in one of four general ways. They (1) fight invaders; (2) promote or regulate normal or desired body functions; (3) slow or stop abnormal or undesired body functions; or (4) provide extra supplies of raw materials needed by the body.

Drugs that combat invading microorganisms (germs) include

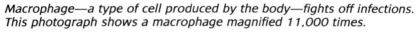

Macrophage—a type of cell produced by the body—fights off infections. This photograph shows a macrophage magnified 11,000 times.

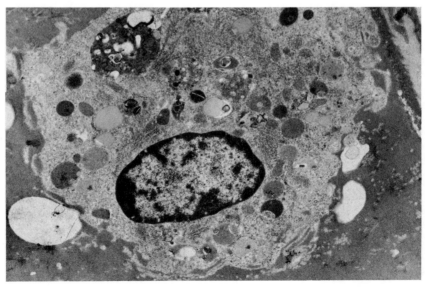

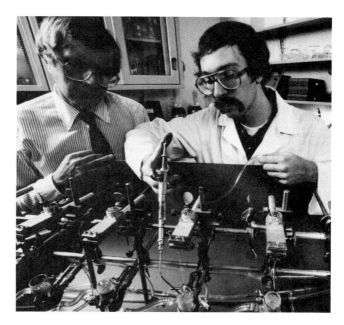

Researchers at a pharmaceutical manufacturer test a vascular-tissue antibiotic, a type of drug that kills or inactivates germs that have already infected the body.

vaccines, which raise the body's defenses so that germs cannot invade it in the first place, and antibiotics, which kill or inactivate germs that have already infected the body. Other anti-infection drugs include antivirals (viruses are germs smaller and more primitive than bacteria and cause flu, chicken pox, and other ills); antiparasiticals (parasites are organisms, such as fleas, that live inside or on the body); and antifungals (a fungus is a mold, such as the one that causes athlete's foot).

A vaccine helps prevent infection by activating the body's immune system (the system that defends the body against invaders) before germs attack instead of after infection has set in, when it may be too late. The vaccine accomplishes this preemptive feat because it contains particles the human body recognizes as disease germs and thus tries to fight off. These particles differ from germs in one important way, however. They cannot cause disease. Instead, they "fool" the immune system into manufacturing antibodies—"defender" cells—that combat germs. Should the body be attacked by influenza germs, for instance, after it has been vaccinated against "the flu," it will have a store of antibodies ready to launch an offensive that will prevent the body from catching the flu.

The second type of drug effect involves the promotion or regulation of normal or desirable body functions. There are hundreds of normal functions the body must accomplish, and hundreds of drugs can aid its efforts. These drugs are often categorized according to the body system they affect. To help the heart do its normal work of pumping blood around the body, for instance, there are cardiac (heart) drugs that make it contract more forcefully, that allow it to fill with blood more completely, that strengthen the electrical impulses that keep it beating regularly, or that keep its vessels relaxed to provide a good blood supply to its own tissues.

Similarly, there are drugs that assist the nervous system by helping nerve impulses move freely along the nerves, for instance. There are also digestive-system drugs that help the body process food. These main-system drug groups may be further divided into subgroups according to the specific way they work on the system.

Because there are so many such categories and because drugs affect the body through so many varieties of interaction, it is not possible to detail them all. But a look at one group, diuretics, reveals in general how drugs can help the body perform one of its normal functions.

A diuretic is a cardiac drug that helps the body rid itself of extra fluid that makes the heart work too hard. One diuretic, the chemical furosemide, works by causing potassium chloride, a chemical normally present in the body, to gather in the kidneys in renal tubules. The potassium chloride located in the tubules makes the body send an excessive amount of water there to dilute the chemical. The extra water flows down the tubules to the bladder and from there is excreted as urine.

As in other cases, the drug's effect depends on an interaction: The diuretic's chemical structure attracts potassium chloride to the kidneys, and the body's normal tendency—to dilute potassium chloride—eventually causes water to leave the body.

The third broad type of drug effect slows or stops unwanted or abnormal body functions. These abnormal functions may be as mild as chapped lips or as serious as cancer. Like drugs used to promote normal function, those used against abnormal body function are often categorized according to the body system that they affect. One undesired body function fought by drugs is pain.

Whatever its cause, whether mild or severe, pain is always

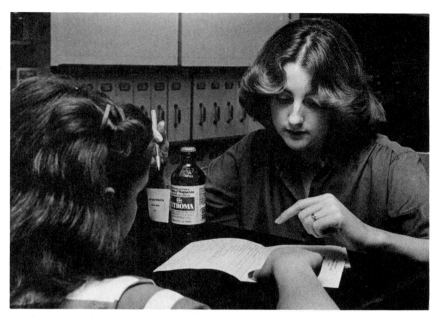

A pharmacist instructs a patient in the proper use of a drug. The printed page they are studying includes medical information not listed on the label of the bottle.

detected, transmitted, and reacted to by parts of the nervous system. Thus, painkillers make up a category of the nervous-system drugs. The drugs can then be divided into even smaller categories, such as general anesthetics (which induce unconsciousness) and narcotics (which cause addiction).

One important member of the narcotic group is morphine, a product of the poppy plant (*Papaver somniferum*). It is not known exactly how morphine acts to relieve pain, but it is known that all narcotics have similar chemical structures and that they resemble enkephalins, the brain's own natural painkilling chemicals. It is generally thought that narcotics attach to "binding sites" in the brain and that the brain mistakes the drug for enkephalins and reacts by turning off pain messages.

Finally, drugs may supply materials the body needs but is not getting in sufficient amounts, such as vitamins and minerals. Some people are undersupplied because their diets are poor; others suffer diseases that prevent the body from extracting important vitamins from food. Oxygen, for example, may be given as a drug to people whose breathing does not furnish an adequate supply of this vital element. In other cases, a drug product provides calories—the "energy" contained in food—to people stricken with an ailment that inhibits normal eating or digestion.

Among the most important materials often furnished through drugs is iron, which the body uses to produce hemoglobin, the part of the red blood cell that carries oxygen to other cells throughout the body. If cells lack sufficient iron, the bone marrow (the spongy tissue inside bones where blood cells are made) makes only small, poorly constructed red cells. The result is iron deficiency anemia, a condition in which small, malformed blood cells cannot perform their crucial oxygen-carrying chores.

Extra iron, often taken in a pill or liquid form, enters the body through the walls of the digestive tract and is eventually deposited in the bone marrow. The marrow immediately uses the iron to make normal blood cells that soon replace the stunted ones. This is one of the simplest kinds of interactive drug effects: The drug supplies a structure (the iron molecule) that the body takes up and uses as a building block.

Whatever purpose is served by a drug, its effects depend on the principle of interaction between the drug and the body. Because drugs are so numerous and the body is so complicated, there are thousands of different interactions that can occur. No matter how the details of such interactions may differ, they all have six basic steps in common. The next chapter examines these six steps more closely and explains in more depth how drugs work.

•   •   •   •

CHAPTER 3

. . . .

HOW DRUGS WORK

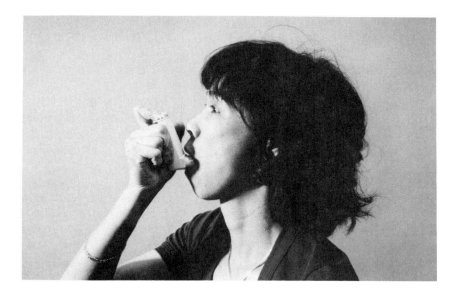

The first step in getting a drug to the place where it can produce its desired effect is administration, that is, giving a drug. The manner in which a drug is given is called its route of administration. Drugs may be inhaled, taken orally (by mouth), injected, or applied to skin or the mucous membrane (skin well-supplied with blood vessels, such as skin in the mouth or nose).

ROUTES OF ADMINISTRATION

Convenience sometimes dictates how a drug is administered. Some people prefer to use nose spray to clear nasal congestion;

others would rather swallow a capsule. More often, however, necessity determines the route of administration because different drugs can enter the bloodstream only in certain ways.

Many drugs can be swallowed—a painless, convenient, and economical route of administration. The trouble is that the drug's action does not begin until it dissolves in the stomach and then is absorbed into the bloodstream; drugs given by other routes enter the blood directly. Also, some drugs irritate the stomach, others taste bad, and some cannot be absorbed through the stomach at all. Certain drugs can be inserted into the rectum, where the mucous membranes take up the drug and distribute it, whereas others work only when injected. Each drug has a most efficient route by which it is absorbed in the right amount and at the right speed.

If a drug cannot be absorbed any other way, or if the body needs the drug to take effect immediately, injection is the best route of administration. Injections may be *subcutaneous* (just under the skin); *intramuscular* (into muscle tissue); *intravenous*

A radiologist draws a chemotherapy drug into a hypodermic needle. Injection is the most efficient route of administration for anticancer drugs.

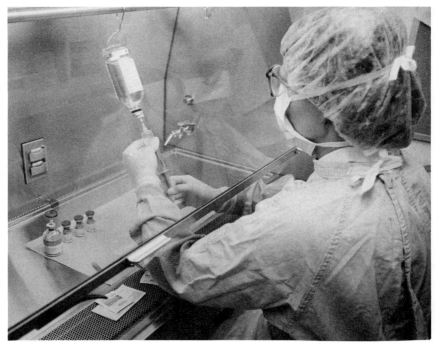

(into a vein); *intra-arterial* (into an artery); or *intradermal* (directly into skin tissue). The type of injection used is often determined by the purpose of the injection. For fast onset of action, for instance, an intravenous injection may be best, whereas a drug meant to reach a certain organ may be injected intra-arterially.

Some drugs can be absorbed from the mucous membrane under the tongue. This *sublingual* (under the tongue) route is often used for the cardiac drug nitroglycerine because such administration is convenient, and action begins rapidly.

Inhalation—breathing in the drug in the form of a gas such as nitrous oxide anesthetic or in an aerosol (a mist of tiny liquid particles)—causes rapid absorption of the drug through the lungs into the blood. Drugs that combat asthma attacks are often administered this way.

Intrathecal administration is the process of injecting a drug directly into the spinal column, where it is distributed by the spinal fluid. Substances are sometimes given intrathecally so that their progress may be tracked on x-ray film.

Topical administration is the application of a drug substance to the skin. Nitroglycerine is sometimes compounded into a paste and administered this way, as are many drugs meant to affect primarily the skin, such as steroid creams used to reduce itching or inflammation.

PROCESSING AND DISTRIBUTION

Once it enters the bloodstream, a drug travels to the liver, the body's "chemical processing plant." The liver breaks the drug down into substances that are less toxic and more easily used by the body. This process, called drug metabolism, involves enzymes—body substances that form chemical reactions with the drug to help break it down. The liver also makes carrier proteins that bind to some of the drug molecules and carry them around the body in the blood. Metabolism is a major part of the transformation step in drug-body interactions.

After the drug has been transformed by the liver, the distribution step occurs. This refers to the process whereby the drug travels in the bloodstream to its site of action, the place where it can do its work. Drug molecules that are not bound to carrier

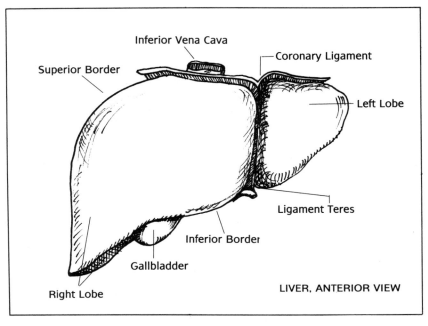

Inferior Vena Cava

Coronary Ligament

Superior Border

Left Lobe

Ligament Teres

Inferior Border

Gallbladder

Right Lobe

LIVER, ANTERIOR VIEW

Once a drug enters the bloodstream it travels to the liver, the "chemical processing plant" that breaks the medication down into substances that the body can use more easily.

proteins travel freely in the blood and bind to receptor sites on the cell itself.

When a drug molecule fills a cell's receptor site, the receptor changes; changes also occur within the cell itself. These changes allow the drug's therapeutic (helpful) effect to take place. There are many varieties of therapeutic effects, including the destruction of disease bacteria, the blockage of pain messages in the brain, an attack on a cancer cell, and others. A branch of medical science, therapeutics, studies the effects of specific drugs.

Drugs do not usually stay inside the body indefinitely. Instead, excess amounts of drug (and by-products formed when the liver breaks the drug down into simpler chemicals) reenter the bloodstream and are excreted, that is, expelled with the body's waste materials, often by the kidneys. The kidneys excrete drugs and by-products by filtering drug-laden blood through *glomeruli*. These membranes send the filtered-out material to the renal tubules, wash the filtrate from the tubules with water, and send the

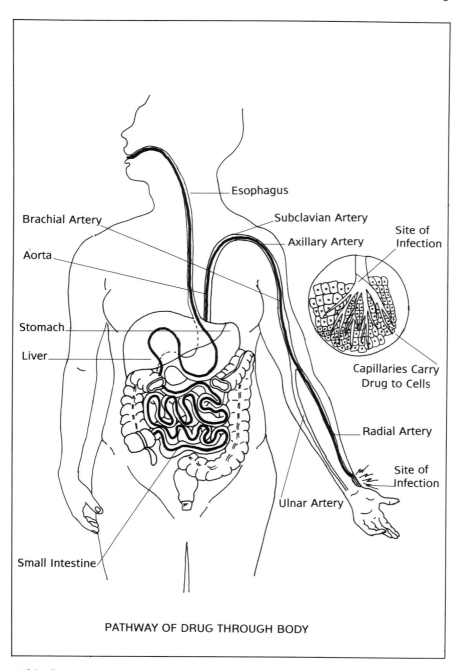

Esophagus

Brachial Artery

Subclavian Artery

Aorta

Axillary Artery

Site of Infection

Stomach

Liver

Capillaries Carry Drug to Cells

Radial Artery

Site of Infection

Ulnar Artery

Small Intestine

PATHWAY OF DRUG THROUGH BODY

This diagram shows the path traveled by food as it passes through the body toward the site of infection, in this instance the patient's wrist.

water on to the bladder. From there the water is excreted as urine. Drugs excreted in solid waste are filtered from the blood by the liver, which includes them in a waste product called bile. The bile flows to a part of the duodenum, moves on to the intestine, and is excreted in the feces, the body's solid waste.

Because the interaction of drug and body is so complex, more than one effect—some therapeutic, some not—can result. Aspirin, for instance, can produce several desired effects. It can decrease pain, lower fever, and reduce inflammation (redness and swelling). But aspirin also has unwanted side effects. It can irritate the stomach and can cause abnormal bleeding by lowering the normal clotting ability of the blood.

FACTORS AFFECTING DRUG ACTION

Many factors influence the effectiveness drugs have on the people who ingest them. One of the most important factors is the patient's own compliance—how well he or she obeys the doctor's instructions for taking the drug properly, regularly, and for the necessary length of time. Some patients may lack the money to buy the drug in the first place or to have it refilled. Others may fail to follow instructions for many reasons, including forgetfulness, anger at the doctor, denial that they are ill, or fear of unpleasant side effects. Sometimes, after a short period of taking the drug, the patient may feel better and decide to discontinue using it, even though, in the long run, halting the use of medications in this way can worsen the person's condition. Even when taken properly, the same drug can affect different people in different ways. One patient may require a greater quantity of painkiller, for instance, than another patient does. This difference, called individual variation, must be assessed by the prescribing physician on a case-by-case basis.

Any drug's action inside the body is affected by how well the medication is absorbed, which in turn depends on the form of the drug itself (some medications are hard tablets; others are liquids); the chemical properties of the drug; and the route of administration. The formulation of a drug—the materials with which a drug's active ingredients are mixed—also affects how well a drug is absorbed. The drug cyclosporine, which helps stop

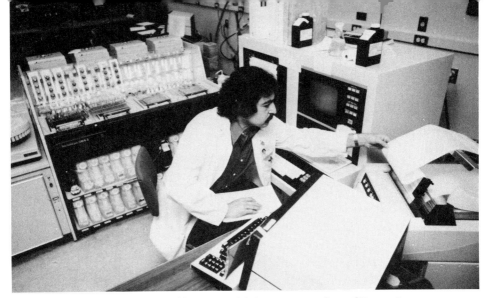

In order for any drug to be effective, a high concentration of it must enter the bloodstream. Here, a cancer researcher uses a computer to analyze the results of blood tests.

the body from rejecting transplanted organs, was initially deemed worthless by researchers. Only when it was mixed in alcohol instead of water did the drug dissolve properly. The mixture was administered orally and afterward appeared in patients' blood samples, proving that formulation is a key to its successful absorption.

Interaction with other drugs may also vary drug effects. Two or more drugs given at the same time may act separately, raise or lower one another's effect, or cause side effects neither would create if given alone. Interaction is one reason why patients should always inform their physician about any other drugs they may be taking.

Some diseases or injuries may raise or lower a drug's effectiveness or cause unusually strong side effects. Patients who have kidney disease, for instance, may experience increased effects and side effects of any drug excreted by the kidneys.

Drug tolerance—getting used to a drug—can decrease a drug's effect. A person addicted to painkilling drugs, for example, will not derive the same pain relief from such medications as will someone who is not addicted, because an addict's body is already used to the presence of the drug.

An obvious factor in determining a drug's effect is dosage. Proper dosages are determined by the manufacturer during tests performed while the drug is in the development stage. These dosage recommendations may then be refined by the prescribing doctor, who takes into account the patient's age, weight, general health, and the surface area of his or her body. The correct dosage of one drug cannot be compared to that of another; for instance, 5 milligrams of the tranquilizer diazepam is about as strong as 100 milligrams of the tranquilizer phenobarbital.

How often the drug is taken crucially affects how well it works. Frequency of dosage is often based on a drug's "half-life," that is, the length of time it takes for half the drug to be excreted from the body. If a drug's half-life is six hours, the patient who takes the drug every six hours will keep a steady amount of the drug in the body, neither so much that toxic effects are caused, nor so little that good effects are lost.

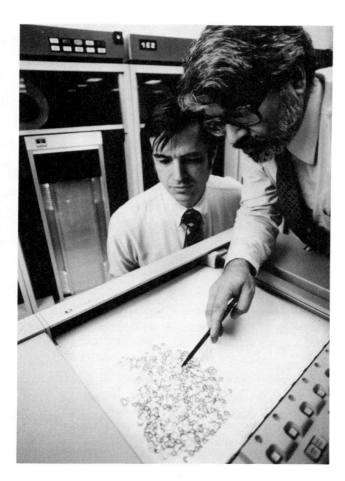

Doctors at Pfizer Inc., a major drug manufacturer, study a computer model of the kidney enzyme renin for clues that may help them develop a drug to combat tension.

A patient's age also alters the effects and side effects of drugs. Infants, for instance, excrete some drugs less efficiently than adults do; thus drugs that are safe for adults can have toxic effects in infants. Elderly persons, too, may excrete drugs less well; thus the elderly may need smaller doses of some drugs than younger people do.

Finally, some inherited factors may influence the way a drug works. People whom scientists call "rapid acetylators" may metabolize (change and excrete) antituberculosis drugs, sulfa drugs, and the anti-high-blood-pressure drug Apresoline faster than other people and so need larger doses. Some people have genetic (inherited) traits that make certain drugs dangerous to them. Those with the inherited disease porphyria, for instance, cannot take certain sedatives because they suffer severe reactions. About 13% of black people and certain whites of Mediterranean ancestry have an enzyme (body chemical) deficiency that makes their blood cells break down when they take the antimalaria drug quinine, some sulfa drugs, and the antibiotics Macrodantin and Furadantin, used to treat bladder infections. This enzyme deficiency can be detected by laboratory tests.

ANTIBIOTICS—A CASE IN POINT

One way to see how the steps of the drug-body interaction occur in real life is to examine the process by which antibiotics work against infection. A doctor treating a cut may observe telltale signs of infection such as pain, redness, swelling, and oozing of infected material. He or she may then culture the wound—take a sample of the infected material to identify the offending bacteria—and then prescribe antibiotic tablets or an antibiotic injection. When the "shot" is given or a tablet swallowed, administration occurs.

Once it reaches the stomach, the tablet dissolves, and its contents are absorbed through the walls of the intestine into the blood. If the drug is given by injection, it reaches the blood directly. Either way, after the drug reaches the liver, drug metabolism occurs, and the blood distributes the drug around the body. Tiny blood vessels at the site of infection bring the drug into contact with bacteria, and therapeutic action begins.

Some antibiotics block the bacteria's ability to form a strong cell wall (cells are the building blocks of living things) by inter-fering with a *mucopeptide*, a molecule in the wall. A cell wall is the bacteria's only "skin"; a weak cell wall makes the bacteria likely to break open, leak out its contents, and die. Drugs that prevent the formation of a strong bacterial cell wall include pen-icillin, cephalosporin, and vancomycin. The bacteria these drugs fight include streptococcus (which causes sore throats), pneu-mococcus (which causes some pneumonias), clostridium (which causes wound infections), and meningococcus (which causes meningitis).

Other antibiotics force bacteria cells to leak their inner con-tents by working themselves into the area between the cell's fat molecules and protein molecules, making the cell walls permeable so that substances can pass through them. Polymyxin is a drug that operates in this manner, and the bacteria it fights include *Salmonella* (which causes food poisoning) and *Pseudomonas* (which causes some wound, lung, and other infections).

Still other antibiotics interfere with the bacteria's protein syn-thesis, its production of proteins that are vital to its life, growth, and reproduction. Antibiotics that stop bacterial protein synthe-sis attach their molecules to the bacteria's ribosomes (protein-making structures) and stop them from performing their task. Drugs that do this include tetracycline, erythromycin, and chlor-amphenicol; they are effective against a wide range of infecting organisms, including those that cause typhus and Rocky Moun-tain spotted fever. Drugs that combat unhealthy yeasts and fungi also disrupt their targets' internal functions. These drugs include nystatin and griseofulvin, used against thrush (a yeast infection of the mouth), ringworm, athlete's foot, and some hair and nail infections. Such drugs also include some of the first anti-infection drugs ever devised—sulfonamides—commonly called sulfa drugs. They prevent bacteria from making folic acid, a substance used to form raw material for new bacteria.

In order for a sufficient amount of any drug to reach the in-fected site, it must first enter the blood in a high concentration. This leads to an excess of the drug that the kidneys later expel. Antibiotics can also have strong side effects on the kidneys, some-times damaging them severely during the process of excretion. Other common antibiotic side effects can include stomach prob-lems, rashes, and fevers. Some of these side effects can be minimized by changing the dose or the route of administration, but sometimes a different drug must be chosen in order to minimize side effects.

Anticancer drugs work very differently from antibiotics, but they interact with the body in roughly the same way. And although there are seven major classes of anticancer drugs, they are all intended to meet a single goal: killing cancer cells while sparing normal cells. One type of anticancer drug is the group of folic acid antagonists, which includes the drug methotrexate. Methotrexate, like other folic acid antagonists, is usually best absorbed into the body by injection. The liver then breaks the drug down into simpler forms, which swim through the bloodstream into every cell, cancerous or not. One of the broken-down forms of methotrexate resembles folic acid so closely that it "fakes out" cells, which will try to use it to make a substance called thymine.

But the attempt fails because the fake folic acid cannot help make thymine. Without thymine, no cell can make DNA, the hereditary material that tells new cells what form to take. As a result, the cell cannot reproduce, and it dies. Folic acid antagonists affect cancer cells sooner than they do normal cells because cancer cells, which reproduce faster, take up the fake folic acid faster. And each cancer cell that dies without reproducing helps kill off the entire cancer.

Folic acid antagonists stop some normal cells from reproducing, however, which explains why methotrexate and many other anticancer drugs have strong side effects. These effects include nausea, vomiting, hair loss, fever, bone aches, blood disorders, lung damage, liver damage, kidney damage, and even death. Yet the drug must be taken in high doses if the cancer is to be fought off effectively. Treating cancer with almost any anticancer drug, in fact, can mean walking a fine line between the dangers of the disease and the risks of treatment.

To reduce the side effects of methotrexate, physicians may recommend a technique called "leucovorin rescue." Leucovorin, a form of folic acid administered to the patient after methotrexate has attacked cancer cells, supplies real folic acid to normal cells before they die, too. (Meanwhile, the methotrexate is excreted by the kidneys; about 90% of the drug is carried out of the body in urine.) Unfortunately, leucovorin rescue cannot altogether eliminate methotrexate's side effects, and the technique can be used only by skilled, experienced cancer specialists who have the proper laboratory equipment for closely monitoring the therapy through blood tests.

As these examples show, the details of exactly how each drug works are complicated and differ from drug to drug. Yet all drugs work according to some general principles, so that even when we do not know precisely how a specific drug works, we can reason out how its effects occur.

•   •   •   •

CHAPTER 4

· · · · · · · · · · · · ·

DOCTOR'S ORDERS

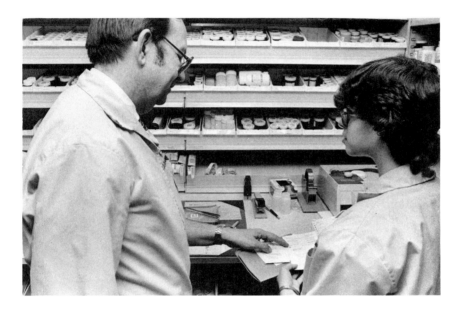

Some drugs are available only through a doctor's prescription, a written order from a physician to a pharmacist authorizing sale of the drug to the patient. Only a licensed physician can legally prescribe drugs, although some medications can be prescribed by dentists, podiatrists (foot doctors), and veterinarians. Only a licensed pharmacist may dispense prescription drugs.

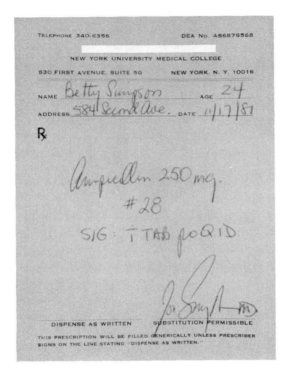

In addition to instructions for the pharmacist, a prescription must include the physician's name, address, signature, medical degree, and—in most states— his or her medical license number (upper right).

Yet, aside from narcotics, which came under legal control in 1914, no drug needed a doctor's order until the U.S. Congress passed the Durham-Humphrey Amendment in 1951. This federal law defined "prescription drugs" as those unsafe for self-medication and required that they be labeled with the legend, "for sale by prescription only." Today, the Food and Drug Administration (FDA) decides whether or not a drug must be designated "prescription only."

The FDA designates a drug as "prescription only" if its effects or side effects are strong enough to pose dangers or if the drug is to be used by people with specific medical problems. The drug Coumadin, for instance, is a prescription drug because its side effects include severe bleeding and because the condition it treats—blood clots—can be so serious that anyone who suffers from it should be under a doctor's care. The painkiller Demerol is a "prescription only" drug because the kinds of pain it relieves often come from conditions that need a doctor's care and also because Demerol can be addictive.

PACKAGE INSERTS

Drug packages must contain a package insert that provides the health professional with detailed facts about the drug. The insert for drug manufacturer Winthrop-Breon's morphine sulfate injections, for instance, describes morphine as a product of opium and morphine sulfate as a white powder that dissolves in water. The manufacturer also includes a drawing of the morphine sulfate molecule, cites the drug's effects and side effects, explains indications for use along with contraindications (circumstances in which the drug should not be used), and explains how to use the drug in a variety of circumstances. The insert next lists precautions that should be taken when morphine is administered and the ways it may interact with other drugs. It warns, as well, that morphine is addictive. The information includes signs and symptoms of, and explains the treatment for, overdosage. Finally, the insert recommends dosages appropriate for adults and children, notes that morphine should not be mixed with certain other drugs, and advises that the drug be kept cool, not frozen, and away from strong light, which may alter its chemical makeup.

As a precaution, physicians generally tell patients some of this information, although often a doctor may decide that certain facts about a drug may unduly frighten the patient and cause harm. But most patients should know something about the drugs they take, such as the drug's name, possible side effects, what to do if side effects occur, what foods or other drugs it may interact with, how much should be taken and how often, what results to expect, and what to do if the patient misses taking a dosage.

Symmetrel (amantadine hydrochloride) has been approved by the FDA as a treatment for certain flu strains. The package insert (next to the bottle) provides useful information to health-care professionals.

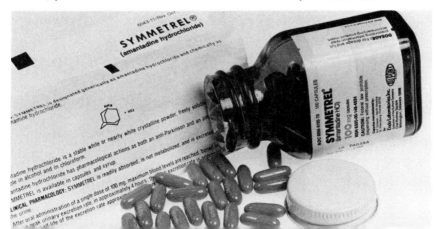

Metric-Apothecary Equivalents

In the United States, physicians choose from two systems of drug measurement. Some use the apothecary system, in which liquid ingredients are measured by minims, drams, ounces, pints, and quarts and dry ingredients are measured in grains and dry ounces. Others follow the metric system, which measures liquid ingredients in liters and milliliters and dry ingredients in grams, milligrams, and micrograms.

The difference between the apothecary and metric systems of drug measurement is usually of practical concern only to the pharmacist, who compounds a mixture according to a doctor's prescription. Conversion from one system to the other is done according to the following table:

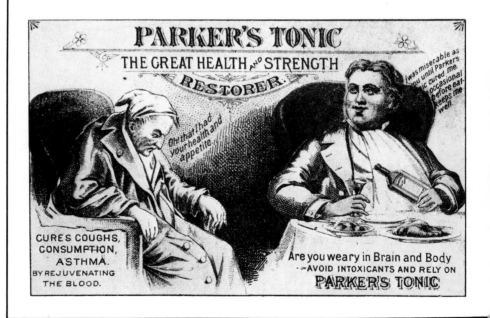

PARKER'S TONIC

THE GREAT HEALTH AND STRENGTH RESTORER.

Oh that I had your health and appetite.

I was miserable as you until Parkers Tonic cured me. I occasional before eat keeps me well

CURES COUGHS, CONSUMPTION, ASTHMA. BY REJUVENATING THE BLOOD.

Are you weary in Brain and Body
AVOID INTOXICANTS AND RELY ON
PARKER'S TONIC

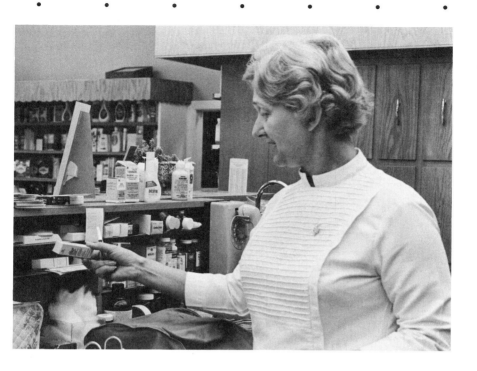

Dry Ingredients

30 grams = 1 ounce
15 grams = 4 drams
10 grams = 2½ drams
7.5 grams = 2 drams
6 grams = 90 grains
750 milligrams = 12 grains
500 milligrams = 7⅕ grains
250 milligrams = 4 grains
125 milligrams = 2 grains
25 milligrams = ⅜ grain
5 milligrams = 1/12 grain
800 micrograms = 1/80 grain
250 micrograms = 1/250 grain
100 micrograms = 1/600 grain

Liquids

1,000 milliliters = 1 quart
750 milliliters = 1½ pints
500 milliliters = 1 pint
250 milliliters = 8 fluid ounces
100 milliliters = 3½ fluid ounces
50 milliliters = 1¾ fluid ounces
30 milliliters = 1 fluid ounce
15 milliliters = 4 fluid drams
(one tablespoon)
10 milliliters = 2½ fluid drams
8 milliliters = 2 fluid drams
5 milliliters = 1¼ fluid drams
(one teaspoon)

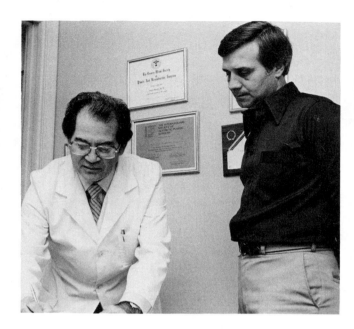

A patient looks on as his doctor writes out a prescription. Most doctors give patients specific instructions about dosage and possible side effects.

THE DOCTOR'S PRESCRIPTION

The doctor's prescription must contain information pertinent to the individual order, including the date it is written, the patient's name, the doctor's name and address, the amount and kind of drug to be given, and the doctor's signature, medical degree, and—in most states—his or her license number. Doctors who prescribe narcotics must add their own federal registration number (which grants them the authority to prescribe controlled drugs) and the patient's address.

The form of a prescription may vary somewhat, but traditionally it consists of four parts:

1. The *superscription*: This is the Rx, an abbreviation for *recipere*, which means "take thou" in Latin.

2. The *inscription*: This is the list of ingredients and their amounts. Because drugs are now often compounded (that is, their ingredients are combined) by manufacturers rather than by pharmacists, the inscription may simply state a product's name as supplied by a drug company.

3. The *subscription*: This is the direction for compounding the drug. Because manufacturers now commonly compound many drugs, the subscription may be brief.

4. The *signature*: This part of the prescription contains the directions to be printed on the label of the drug container; for example, "Take one tablet twice daily, in the morning and at bedtime."

Other items may appear on a prescription because they aid the patient or the pharmacist. Knowing the patient's age, for instance, enables the pharmacist to confirm that the dosage is correct. Pharmacists also find it helpful to know how many refills the patient should be allowed. (Refills of narcotics are regulated by federal law; whereas some may not be refilled, others may be refilled five times in the six months following the doctor's original order.) Other useful information includes instructions that tell the pharmacist how to label the container so that the drug may be identified rapidly in case the patient suffers allergy, overdose, or side effects. A wealth of prescription information also is of use to a new physician—in the event the patient changes doctors.

Finally, if the ordered drug is available from more than one manufacturer, the prescription may either direct the pharmacist to give only a certain product or allow the pharmacist to choose a preferred manufacturer. The choice is often between a product made by the company that first developed and sold the drug (the "brand name" drug) and the same substance made into a drug

(continued on page 56)

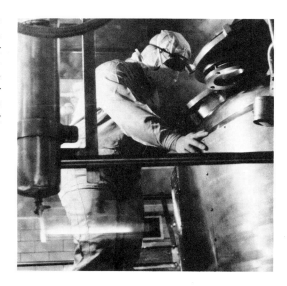

A worker employed by a drug manufacturer operates a mixing tank that produces penicillin. Federal regulations require drug workers to wear protective clothing to guard them in the event of a dangerous mishap.

Pharmacy Careers

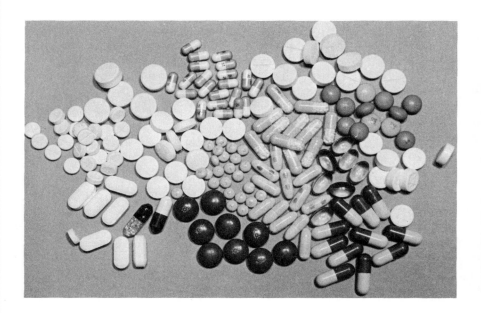

There are three major types of professional pharmacy careers. The most highly educated pharmacy professionals are pharmacologists, scientists who employ a wide range of scientific knowledge to find and develop drugs. Clinical pharmacologists study the prop- erties of drugs and their effects on the human body. Toxicologists study poisonous materials and ex- plore ways to minimize their harmful effects on living orga- nisms. Biochemical pharmacolo- gists study the way drugs interact with the minute mechanisms located inside the body's cells. There are also a number of other special areas on which pharmacologists may concentrate.

Pharmacologists work in drug companies, in hospitals, at universities and foundations, or in government or industry. They must have a college degree with a strong emphasis in science, plus a doctorate in pharmacology (normally this involves four or five years of postgraduate study). Professionals in this field may also have a medical degree, which takes another four years to earn. Some schools give combined Ph.D-M.D. degrees. Because they do not dispense drugs to the public, pharmacologists need not be licensed, certified, or registered by state or federal governments.

Pharmacists provide the link between pharmacology and the public. They are knowledgeable about drug composition, effects and side effects, and know the best ways of administering drugs

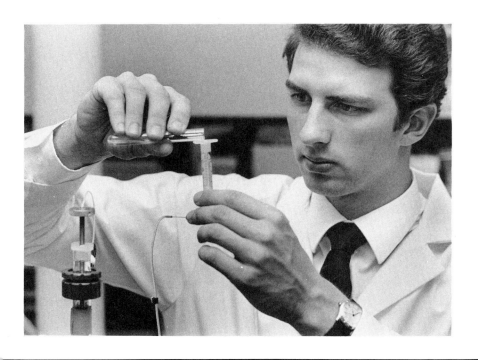

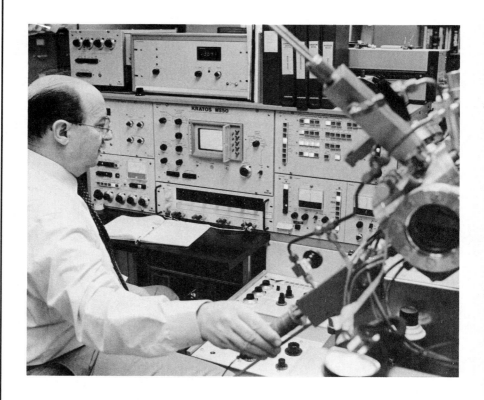

under different circumstances. Like pharmacologists, pharmacists are highly educated. They must have a college degree heavily weighted toward science and must complete either a five-year program leading to a degree in pharmacy or a six-year program leading to a Doctor of Pharmacy (Pharm. D.). Because pharmacists dispense drugs to the general public all states require them to be licensed. Most states also require pharmacists to practice under the supervision of experienced pharmacists before striking out on their own.

Pharmacists work in many possible settings, from the corner drugstore to the hospital pharmacy; they may also teach in nursing, medical, and pharmacy schools. In addition to acquiring knowledge about drugs, many pharmacists take business courses because they often run stores that stock a variety of nondrug products.

A pharmacy technician is a professional pharmacist's helper. Pharmacy technicians relieve pharmacists of many routine tasks related to preparing and dispensing drugs. They type labels, inventory drug stocks, and handle other clerical tasks. They may also deliver drugs from central storage to areas where the drugs are used, such as from hospital pharmacies to floors where patients are located. They are usually required to complete college courses in science and math. They may be trained on the job by a pharmacist or may take a two-year course leading to an associate's degree in pharmacy technology.

Pharmacy technicians are often employed in hospitals and other large health-care facilities. They are not required to be licensed or certified because they do not dispense drugs directly to the public, but they may be required to have such credentials at some time in the future. Pharmacy technicians usually cannot advance much from fairly low-level "helper" jobs unless they return to school to get more advanced formal education in pharmacy.

Upon entering the profession, every pharmacist takes the following oath:

At this time, I vow to devote my professional life to the service of mankind through the profession of pharmacy.

I will consider the welfare of humanity and relief of human suffering my primary concerns.

I will use my knowledge and skills to the best of my ability in serving the public and other health professionals.

I will do my best to keep abreast of developments and maintain professional competency in my profession of pharmacy.

I will obey the laws governing the practice of pharmacy and will support enforcement of such laws.

I will maintain the highest standards of moral and ethical conduct.

I take these vows voluntarily with the full realization of the trust and responsibility with which I am empowered by the public.

(continued from page 51)
product by another company (the "generic" drug), often at a lower cost. But there is yet another type of prescription that a doctor may issue if he or she had received authorization—a prescription for one of the drugs in the group known as controlled drugs.

CONTROLLED DRUGS

Some drugs are considered so dangerous or have such high potential for abuse that they are regulated by special federal laws. Doctors who prescribe such drugs—controlled drugs—must apply for permission to do so. They then receive a federal registration number that appears on every prescription they write for the substance. Doctors must renew their registration annually.

Dangerous drugs or those that can potentially be abused are categorized by schedules geared to the level of danger they present.

Schedule I drugs include substances forbidden for use except under research conditions by qualified scientists, who must obtain clearance from the FDA. These drugs include marijuana, LSD, and heroin.

Schedule II drugs also have a high potential for abuse but are accepted for use in treatment. This category includes strong painkillers such as morphine, potent tranquilizers, and cocaine. Physicians who have registration numbers may prescribe these drugs once for a patient but they cannot order refills nor prescribe over the telephone. The U.S. Department of Justice regulates the total quantity of Schedule II drugs manufactured in the United states.

Schedule III drugs—one such is the painkiller codeine—are also dangerous but have less potential for abuse than those listed in Schedules I and II.

Schedule IV drugs—for instance, the painkiller Darvon—resemble those listed in Schedule III. The main difference is that illegal possession of Schedule IV drugs carries a lesser penalty.

Schedule V drugs include exempt narcotics—drugs that seldom are abused although they have some potential for abuse. A doctor dispensing any of these drugs must keep a record of the prescription for two years. Schedule V drugs include Lomotil, an antidiarrhea drug, and some compounds containing very small amounts of codeine.

BRAND NAME VERSUS GENERIC

Unless a physician requests no substitutions on a prescription, pharmacists in all 50 states may dispense generic rather than brand name drugs. This can mean big savings for the consumer. Yet controversy surrounds some substitutions for reasons that are clear to those who know something about how drugs are named, patented, and sold by companies that first develop them.

When a drug company discovers or develops a new drug substance, it obtains a patent for the substance and sometimes also for the process of manufacturing it. A patent is a form of legal protection that gives the patent owner exclusive control of the patented item for 17 years. The drug substance furosemide, for example, was developed by Hoechst-Roussel Pharmaceuticals, Inc. In 1962, while the drug was undergoing tests to get the FDA's approval, the company patented furosemide. So until 1979 only Hoechst-Roussel was allowed to make and sell furosemide. This is accepted as a fair practice because it costs companies a great deal of money—sometimes more than $90 million—to get a drug past the FDA approval stage and on the market. Once a new drug reaches the market, though, it may earn $200 to $300 million per year for its company as long as it remains under patent protection. Once Hoechst-Roussel passed the FDA's tests, it earned back the expense of developing the drug and reaped a considerable profit.

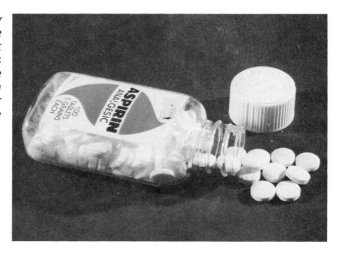

Aspirin is one of many remedies that can be purchased in generic forms. Generics are as effective as brand name drugs but cost less, often because the manufacturer avoids the expense of fancy packaging.

These profits were sure to dwindle, however, as soon as the patent expired. Hoechst-Roussel prepared for this contingency by giving the drug a registered trade name that would never expire. The company called the drug Lasix, which is shorter and easier to remember than furosemide. Hoechst-Roussel hoped that even when other companies began making furosemide, patients would remember the trade name Lasix and prefer it to whatever competitors' products emerged.

In 1979, when the furosemide patent expired, other companies received FDA approval to make and sell the drug. Ever since, furosemide has been available under the brand name Lasix, made only by Hoechst-Roussel, and under its generic name, furosemide, from other companies. But although the drug's makers all use the active ingredient furosemide, they do not all use the same process or the same "inert ingredients"—the capsule or tablet coating and the filler material that makes up most of a capsule or other drug form—when compounding a drug.

By 1987, more than 70 drug companies were making generic furosemide. They sold their products more cheaply to make them attractive to people who had been using Lasix. They could afford to do so because they had not borne the costs of developing the drug (shouldered by Hoechst-Roussel), nor did they spend huge sums on advertising its effectiveness. But was generic furosemide as safe and effective as Hoechst-Roussel's original product, Lasix?

The FDA maintains that every generic drug it approves—a total of some 5,000 as of 1987—is as safe and effective as its brand name equivalent. To get FDA approval, a generic must contain the same active ingredients as the original drug, be given in the same dosage, have the same dosage form (tablet, syrup, and so on), and have the same route of administration. It must also be bioequivalent, that is, it must get into the body in about the same amount of time and at about the same speed and work as effectively as the brand name drug.

Brand name manufacturers sometimes hold that even FDA-approved generics do not always satisfy this last requirement. These manufacturers point to an element that helps determine bioequivalence, bioavailability, the measurement of how much drug gets into the body and how fast. Bioavailability depends on many things: A tablet's hardness or coating, for instance, can affect how quickly it dissolves in the stomach; different inert ingredients may change the rate at which the drug is absorbed. The FDA allows generic bioavailability to vary by plus or minus 20%, which can amount to a serious difference in the effectiveness of some drugs, according to brand name manufacturers. FDA scientists counter that 20% is not usually enough to change effectiveness or safety. They add that although a 20% difference is legal, the difference that actually occurs is only about 3.5% and that only a few drugs have such narrow safety ranges that a 3.5% difference in bioavailability can pose problems. These drugs include the heart drug digoxin (Lanoxin), the hormone levothyroxine (Synthroid, Levothroid), and the blood-thinning drug warfarin (Coumadin).

Meanwhile, a recent consumer magazine survey found that the 11 most frequently prescribed drugs cost 70% more in their brand name form than in the generic form. In 1985 the Federal Trade Commission (FTC) said generic drugs saved consumers $236 million. And in 1987 the U.S. Department of Health and Human Services (HHS) said federal health-aid programs would pay only for the cheaper generics as long they were found to be effective by consulting physicians.

Brand name manufacturers have claimed that this policy is unfair because it slights companies that have borne the staggering costs of finding and developing the drugs. Even without losing the business the HHS has funneled toward generic companies, brand name manufacturers see their profits tumble as soon as competition from generic-drug makers hits the marketplace. When the patent on the antibiotic Garamycin expired in 1981, its sales dropped by 58%. Brand name companies say that continued reductions in their profits will discourage them from spending a fortune on developing new drugs. Why should they, when other companies can step in and reap the benefits of cheap imitations?

Doctors and pharmacists, meanwhile, are caught in the middle. They want to dispense safe, effective drugs at the lowest cost, but they tend to favor brand names because they are familiar with them through the drug companies' advertising campaigns. (The FDA says brand name companies spend $4 billion per year promoting their drug products.) Doctors and pharmacists claim they are not swayed so much by advertising as by their preference for using products that have proved reliable in the past. A 1985 FTC survey found that if given a choice between brand name and generic, pharmacists prescribe generics only 15% of the time, unless they are asked to do otherwise.

For ordinary patients in search of effective drugs, this controversy may be confusing. But patients should remember that they have every right to inform their physician that they prefer a safe, effective form of drug at the most economical cost. In cases when generic drugs are not appropriate, the doctor will say so. Patients should also ask their doctor any other questions that occur to them about drugs; knowledge about prescription drugs—brand name and generic alike—remains our best possible tool for taking them safely and effectively.

•　　　•　　　•　　　•

CHAPTER 5

· · · · · · · · · · · · · · · · ·

OVER-THE-COUNTER DRUGS

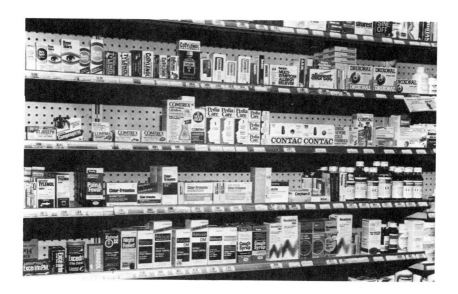

O ver-the-counter (OTC) drugs are medications that a person can buy without a doctor's prescription. There is a huge variety of such products, including remedies for acne, cold symptoms, upset stomach, headache, and many others. Indeed, in the United States, 300,000 OTC drug products containing 800 active ingredients are on the market, and the American Medical Association (AMA) has estimated that 75% of all symptoms are treated with such remedies.

Because these drugs are legal and can be bought without a

doctor's prescription, it may seem that they must also be safe and effective. But, in fact, OTC drugs can be harmful. Some cause allergic reactions. Others interact badly with prescription drugs that patients are also taking. Still others mask serious symptoms that should be treated by a doctor. Moreover, in some cases, OTC drug products prove entirely ineffective or unsafe.

THE FDA AND DRUG REVIEW

Some OTC drugs now available in the United States have not been reviewed by the FDA for safety or effectiveness. The reason is that only since 1938 has federal law required OTC drug makers to establish the safety of new products. Many products sold before 1938 never had to provide such proof, and some of them remain on the market today. Moreover, drugs that have been proved safe through testing can still be harmful to consumers. And even safe OTC drugs may not be effective, because the FDA has required effectiveness tests only since 1962.

In 1962 the FDA began to check the safety and effectiveness of drugs that had entered the marketplace before the days of mandatory testing. These new tests produced shocking results. Of the first 500 products studied, 75% were found either unsafe or ineffective for one or more of their intended uses. Fifteen years later the situation had improved, as FDA action had forced some

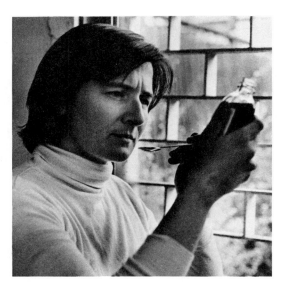

Anyone taking an OTC drug should read the label carefully. Even a seemingly harmless remedy such as cough syrup usually contains ingredients that may cause a bad reaction.

OTC-drug makers to take ineffective or unsafe drugs off drugstore shelves.

Among the drugs the FDA removed from OTC sale were those containing camphorated oil, an ointment that caused many accidental poisonings, and hexachlorophene, once a common ingredient in soaps but now believed to damage the nervous system, especially in infants. Two whole categories of OTC drugs, daytime sedatives (which combat nervousness) and oral wound-healing products, were removed from the market altogether because there was insufficient evidence of their safety and effectiveness.

Labels on many OTC drugs also had to be changed to conform with current FDA rules. Products meant to prevent sunburn, for instance, now must cite the remedy's sun protection factor (SPF). Labels on OTC drugs must also include warnings. Thus, any OTC whose drug ingredient is absorbed into the body must bear a label reading: "As with any drug, if you are pregnant or nursing a baby, seek the advice of a health professional before using this product." When an OTC product is known to interact with other drugs the consumer might be taking, this fact also must appear; some antacids, for example, must bear labels warning that they may reduce the effects of tetracycline, an antibiotic.

As of 1988, a great deal still remained to be done to guarantee the effectiveness and safety of all OTC drugs. In fact, only 21 of 81 FDA-established categories for OTC drugs had finished their FDA tests. Among the OTC categories that had been completely tested were antacids, bronchodilators (asthma remedies), cough remedies, and eardrops. In the case of the other 63 categories, some of the drugs had not yet been tested and some results had not yet been evaluated. Nonetheless, these OTC products remained on drugstore shelves. Until the FDA has reviewed all the ingredients in all 81 OTC drug categories, consumers must continue to test most OTC drugs for themselves.

KEY DECISIONS

Many people mistakenly think they can get all the information they need about OTC drugs from advertisements. Ads, however, are meant not to educate consumers but to sell products. An advertisement for an antiacne skin cream, for instance, may include a picture of a pretty, clear-skinned young woman with

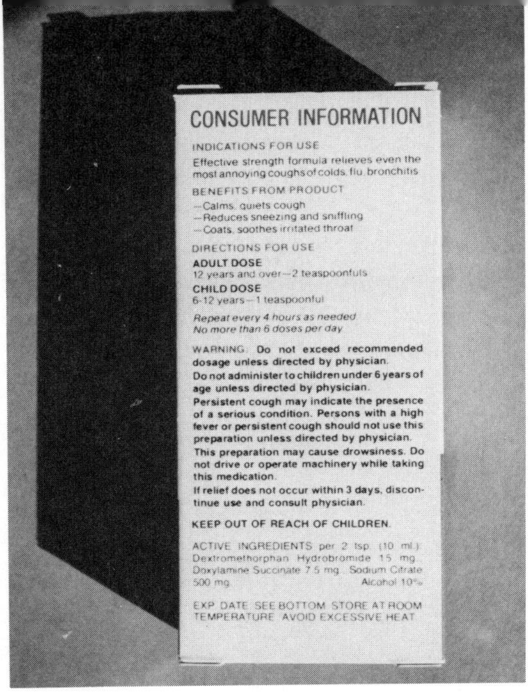
CONSUMER INFORMATION
INDICATIONS FOR USE
Effective strength formula relieves even the most annoying coughs of colds, flu, bronchitis
BENEFITS FROM PRODUCT
—Calms, quiets cough
—Reduces sneezing and sniffling
—Coats, soothes irritated throat
DIRECTIONS FOR USE
ADULT DOSE
12 years and over—2 teaspoonfuls
CHILD DOSE
6-12 years—1 teaspoonful
Repeat every 4 hours as needed
No more than 6 doses per day
WARNING: Do not exceed recommended dosage unless directed by physician.
Do not administer to children under 6 years of age unless directed by physician.
Persistent cough may indicate the presence of a serious condition. Persons with a high fever or persistent cough should not use this preparation unless directed by physician.
This preparation may cause drowsiness. Do not drive or operate machinery while taking this medication.
If relief does not occur within 3 days, discontinue use and consult physician.
KEEP OUT OF REACH OF CHILDREN.
ACTIVE INGREDIENTS per 2 tsp. (10 ml.): Dextromethorphan Hydrobromide 15 mg., Doxylamine Succinate 7.5 mg., Sodium Citrate 500 mg. Alcohol 10%
EXP DATE SEE BOTTOM. STORE AT ROOM TEMPERATURE. AVOID EXCESSIVE HEAT.

Current FDA regulations specify the information that must be included on the label of OTC drugs. The manufacturer's warning is prominently featured on this cold remedy.

several young men vying for her attention. Such an ad appeals to our desires but avoids the issues of effectiveness and safety, which are results of the drug's active ingredients and how they interact with the body.

Rather than rely on the claims made by an ad, consumers should pose the following simple questions when they are about to purchase an OTC drug:

1. What symptoms do I want to remedy with this product, and what is causing the symptoms? This question clarifies a key difference between prescription and OTC drugs. In general, prescription drugs work against causes of symptoms—against the conditions that produce discomfort. OTC drugs, in general, work only against the symptoms themselves. Knowing exactly what symptom needs relief, identifying its cause, and making sure it is not a condition that ought to be treated by a physician—these are the first things to think about when considering use of an OTC remedy.

2. Will the ingredients in this product work effectively against my particular symptoms? Aspirin, ibuprofen, and acetaminophen—all OTC pain relievers—are generally safe and effective. Aspirin and acetaminophen also reduce fever

symptoms, but ibuprofen does not. So for pain and fever symptoms, aspirin or acetaminophen may be better choices. On the other hand, ibuprofen often works better than aspirin or acetaminophen against menstrual cramping. Knowing what an OTC drug can and cannot do is of crucial importance in deciding which OTC drug—if any—to purchase and use.

3. Is this product safe for me to take? To answer this question, read the label. According to James Grogan, director of pharmacy services at St. Louis State Hospital College of Pharmacy, of all the patients who require hospitalization for drug-related reasons some 20% are suffering reactions to OTC drugs. In many cases, these reactions could have been avoided if the victim had investigated safety questions before buying and taking the drug. People allergic to aspirin, for example, may also be allergic to ibuprofen, and ibuprofen labels say so. Anyone with a condition listed in the "Warnings" or "Contraindications" sections of OTC drug labels should not take the product. A major cause of problems in OTC drugs is al-

The poison-control center stickers on these OTC drugs include a phone number consumers can call if the medication causes a bad reaction.

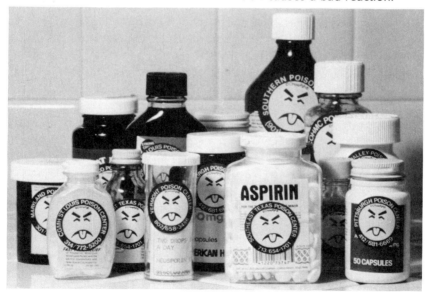

cohol, which is used as an ingredient in more than 500 different products. No alcoholic should use any of these products, even though they may be safe for anyone else.

4. What possible side effects does the product have, and am I prepared to handle them? Some OTC products that are designed to combat cold symptoms, for instance, may cause drowsiness. This is not a problem for someone who intends to stay home getting rest and drinking plenty of fluids—the recommended treatment for a cold. But for someone who must drive a car, operate machinery, or care for small children, drowsiness may be hazardous. Gauging the side effects an OTC drug may cause under specific circumstances is an important consideration for every consumer about to purchase a remedy. A person who takes prescription medications must also know whether or not the OTC drug will interact with the prescription drug. The best way to find out is to check with a doctor or pharmacist.

Generic OTC drugs present another area of concern for the consumer. Sometimes several OTC companies make similar products that contain the same active ingredients to fight the same symptoms. The brand-name drug may be made by a well-known company, whereas the generic drug is a cheaper, less advertised copy. Or there may be two or more well-known brand name makers in addition to generic manufacturers.

In such cases, remember that attractive ads and packages do nothing to relieve symptoms. The FDA requires generic OTC drug products to be manufactured in a similar way to brand name products, to contain the same ingredients, and to be equally effective. The pain-relief drug ibuprofen, for example, may be available in shiny tablets that are advertised on television or in plain-looking tablets from a drug company that saves money by not advertising at all. Both are ibuprofen, though the difference in cost may amount to $3 or $4 per 50 tablets. Someone who is uncertain about the merit of a generic OTC product should consult a pharmacist.

•   •   •   •

CHAPTER 6

A DOSE OF
DISCOVERY

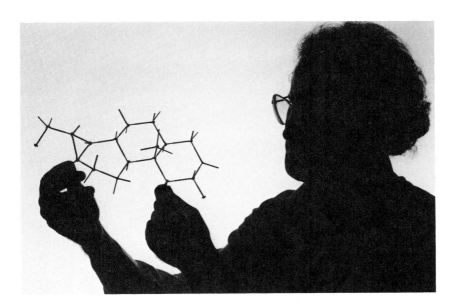

"Each drug has its own way of being born," says drug research scientist and executive Clement Stone, senior vice-president for the research laboratory operated by the drug company Merck Sharp & Dohme. And the birth of each new drug comes only after a long, difficult process.

Consider that just finding substances that will potentially make good medicines can take ten years or longer. When scientists at Merck Sharpe & Dohme began their search for a drug that would lower levels of cholesterol (a substance that can clog arteries and cause heart attacks), they first spent 20 years studying how the body makes and gets rid of cholesterol. In doing so, they found more than 20 previously unknown chemical reactions that occur inside the body.

Why was so much preliminary study necessary? In the words of drug researcher Rhoda Gruen, a biochemist at Hoffman-La Roche drug company, "Diseases are complex. If you want to intervene in the disease . . . you try to break it down into its parts. You then analyze those parts to find out what abnormal events are occurring" in the body's cells.

STAGES OF TESTING

Simply put, researchers must know what is wrong before they try to fix it. Finding out more about how the body works—both when healthy and when ill—is one basic step in drug research. The next basic step is the search for and perfection of drugs that can alter the body's workings and restore malfunctions back to their proper functioning. On average, drug companies spend about $65 million to find and develop a new drug and $60 million more getting it from the laboratory to the marketplace. Hoffman-

A magnified cross section of an abnormally hardened and thickened arterial wall, a symptom of heart disease.

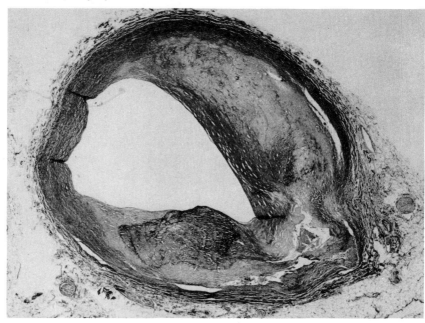

La Roche, a drug company whose sales in the United States total more than $1 billion per year, spends about $2 million per day on international drug research.

The Search for Substances

Once scientists have identified that facet of a disease process they want to attack, they begin looking for promising substances. Researchers conduct test-tube experiments, called assays, in which they add chemicals to laboratory-grown cells in order to find a chemical that has some effect on living tissue. They use computers to simulate the disease and to design drugs that might work against it. They search the natural world of viruses, fungi, and molds to find one that makes a product that fights the disease. The search may lead them to test 100,000 different organisms. If an effective substance is found, the research moves on to the next stage, testing the drug on animals.

Animal Testing

The purpose of animal testing is to learn whether a drug has toxic side effects and to determine the safety of various dosages. Tests show how much drug gets into the animal's blood, how it is broken down by the body, and how the drug is excreted.

One important measurement is the absorption rate—how much drug gets into the animal's blood and how fast. "If the drug's active ingredients don't get into the blood, it won't work," said Ronald Kuntzman, Hoffman-La Roche's vice president for research and development, in an interview that appeared in *New Drug Development in the United States*, an FDA publication issued in January 1988. Scientists search for drugs with high absorption rates so that patients can take them in small amounts, which lessens the likelihood of bad side effects.

By this stage in the process, many new drugs have already been rejected by scientists because they are unsafe, poorly absorbed, or ineffective. In fact, only about 10% of all new drugs end up showing any promise at all, and only about 1% ever come to be tested on human beings. Fewer than 1 in 2,000 of all drugs tested are eventually judged safe and effective enough to be approved for sale.

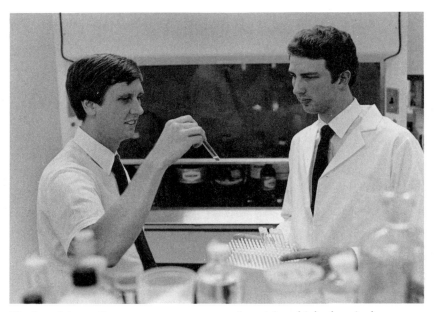

Biochemists perform an assay, an experiment in which chemicals are added to cells grown in a test tube. If a chemical produces the desired effect on the cells, it will then be tested on living tissue.

Testing in Humans

Once a drug reaches the human test stage, strict rules control the process. Scientists who want to test a drug on humans must apply for permission from the FDA through a form called an Investigational New Drug Application. If the FDA agrees the drug is safe enough for experimental use on people, scientists can initiate clinical trials. If the drug is meant for treatment of a rare disease, which means only a small market will exist for it but that for a few patients the drug will prove of great value, the FDA may classify it as an "orphan drug" and give the drug company special testing incentives and tax benefits. This compensates the company for spending a lot of money on a drug that has little potential for profit.

The Three Phases

Clinical trials occur in three phases. In phase 1, researchers learn more about the safety of the drug by administering it to fewer than 100 healthy volunteers. This phase often lasts six months to one year. About 70% of all the drugs that enter this first phase of clinical trials are shown to be safe in doses strong enough to be possibly effective. These drugs enter phase 2.

In phase 2, a few hundred patients receive experimental treatment with the new drug at the same time that others are given either the standard treatment for their disease or a placebo (an inactive substance). Often these tests are "blind studies" (neither the patients nor the scientists know who is getting the test drug and who is not). Blind studies make sure that scientists' hopes for the test drug do not affect the conclusions they draw from the test results. The main purpose of phase 2 trials is to learn more about a drug's effectiveness.

Patients who volunteer to take part in phase 2 clinical trials of new drugs act as "human guinea pigs." They may be doing so because no effective treatment for their disease currently exists and a new drug is their only hope. Other volunteers may hope the new drug will work better than the treatment they are currently receiving or feel that although the drug is unlikely to help them, it may someday help someone else. But whatever motives patients may have, the FDA requires that scientists design the tests rigorously, inform the patients about the possible risks and benefits of the tests, and perform the tests ethically—that is, to respect the volunteers' rights.

The FDA requires institutional review boards (IRBs) to watch over the rights and safety of test volunteers at hospitals where phase 2 clinical trials occur. Review-board members include doctors, scientists, and other experts, including at least one non-scientist, such as a lawyer or minister, and at least one person not affiliated with the hospital where the tests are being done. The board makes sure that the test volunteers give informed consent (which means that they understand the possible risks and benefits of the tests and are volunteering freely); that the volunteers face the fewest possible risks; that they are not subjected to needless pain or discomfort; that results are monitored to make sure the tests proceed safely; and that the volunteers' privacy is maintained. Also, patients must be told they are free to quit the study at any time, for any reason, and that their decision to leave will not affect the care their physicians give them. Volunteers who elect to continue then enter phase 3 clinical trials.

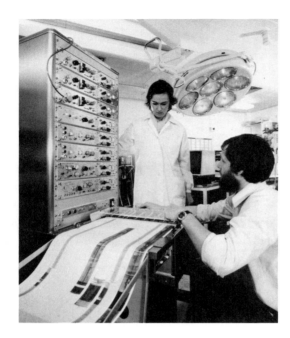

Drug researchers use a polygraph recorder, which measures cardio-vascular function, in their search for new stimulants that may help people stricken with heart disease.

Clinical Trials and Controversy

In spite of careful regulation, clinical trials remain controversial. Some people argue that giving placebos as part of clinical trials is unethical, especially when the volunteers are afflicted with mortal ills. They say that in such cases all the volunteers should be given the new drug, not an inactive substance, because the new drug offers at least the hope of improvement.

But to do so would make the trials much less useful; a strong reason for testing in the first place is to find out if the tested drug is better than nothing. Researchers add that testing a new drug against a placebo allows the new drug to become available to more people more quickly. In 1985 trials of the anti-AIDS drug zidovudine, for example, the drug worked so well when measured against a placebo that further trials were suspended. Instead, Burroughs-Welcome, the drug's manufacturer, asked the FDA to make an exception to the trial regulations. Patients receiving zidovudine were clearly living longer, so it would be unethical not to give all patients in the study this life-prolonging medicine. The FDA agreed. Phase 3 trials were bypassed altogether, and zidovudine was approved for marketing in only four months. In short, because a placebo was used in the phase 2 trials, the new drug, now marketed as Retrovir, reached many patients very quickly.

The zidovudine experience helped the FDA realize that a faster way was needed to get new drugs to very sick people. "There are times," says FDA commissioner Dr. Frank Young, ". . . when a new drug shows so much promise that it would be cruel to withhold it."

Thus, in 1987 the FDA formally permitted drugs that may help desperately ill patients to bypass the usual testing through "fast tracking." To qualify for fast tracking, a drug that has entered phase 2 of clinical trials can be sped through the remainder of the process as long as it has been shown to be safe and possibly effective. For serious, non-life-threatening illnesses, new drugs must usually complete phase 3 of the clinical trial before the FDA approves them for wider use, but they are still available sooner than drugs intended for use against nonserious diseases.

Winning Approval

Drugs that enter phase 3 trials—and only about 25% of drugs entering clinical trials reach this stage—are tested on thousands of patients. The purpose is to acquire knowledge that will enable the drug to be used properly. Phase 3 tests reveal rare side effects, disclose more of the drug's risks and benefits, and provide information that physicians need if they are to prescribe the drug safely and effectively.

The duration of phase 3 trials differs according to how the drug is meant to be used. Antibiotics that will only be taken for a few days or weeks may complete the phase in two years, whereas medications that patients must take for the rest of their lives must be tested for long-term effects. "There are very few illnesses that can't be made worse" by an insufficiently tested drug, says Dr. Young. "Risks and benefits must be measured carefully."

Once phase 3 trials are completed, the drug company asks the FDA for permission to sell the new drug. The company submits a New Drug Application (NDA) that relays all the information the drug company has gained about the new substance. Within 180 days, FDA scientists review the information and decide whether the drug company's results establish the safety and effectiveness of the new drug. If the results pass muster, the drug is approved for sale. The whole process, from discovery to market, may take as few as 3 years or as many as 20.

Orphan Drugs

Sometimes drug companies spend a great deal of money and effort on drugs that are useful only to people who suffer from very rare diseases. The FDA's office of Orphan Products identifies new drugs for rare diseases and provides financial benefits to drug companies that agree to develop and market such drugs. The FDA also provides guidelines to help investigators speed testing, makes outright grants of sums ranging from $20,000 to $70,000 to support the costs of testing, and speeds the drugs' eventual approval process. In this way victims of rare diseases can get new treatments for their ailments, and drug makers can afford to spend money developing the drugs.

The orphan drugs that have been developed under the Office of Orphan Products include trientine. Only about 100 people needed this drug in 1982, but it saved their lives. They had Wilson's disease, an ailment that prevents the body from excreting copper. Only 8,000 people in the United States had the fatal ailment when trientine was discovered; of these, 100 could not tolerate the usual treatment for Wilson's disease and needed trientine to survive. With incentives from the government, the drug company Merck Sharpe & Dohme took on the costly job of testing trientine and bringing it to market. Thus the new drug became available to people who needed it to save their lives.

Other drugs developed through the orphan drug process include

- Pentamidine isethionate, which treats pneumonias that strike victims of immune-system diseases.
- Digoxin-specific antibody fragments, which treat life-threatening overdoses of the cardiac drug digoxin.
- Clofazimine, which combats a form of leprosy.
- Alpha-fetoprotein, which tests the effectiveness of certain cancer treatments.
- Naltrexone, which treats some drug addictions.
- Cyclosporine, which suppresses the immune system so the body will not reject transplanted organs.

- Desmopressin, which treats hemophilia, a disorder in which blood fails to clot.
- Etoposide, an anticancer drug.

The Constant Vigil

Even after a new drug reaches the market, the FDA continues to monitor it, and for two main reasons. First, some side effects do not show up until after doctors have begun prescribing the remedy. Second, once a drug becomes available, doctors may prescribe it for uses other than those for which it was originally intended. The blood-pressure drug minoxidil, for example, turned out to cause hair growth in bald men and began to be used for that purpose. Naltrexone, a drug used to treat heroin addiction, turned out to be useful against Kaposi's sarcoma, a cancer that plagues some AIDS patients. Thus, many new drugs end up being used by patients who may react differently from

These medicine labels advise patients to follow precautions when taking certain drugs.

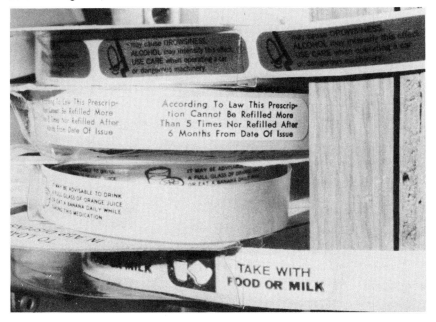

test patients. If problems arise for these new patients, the FDA alerts doctors and the public, requires label changes, or may order the drug withdrawn from the market.

We can take prescribed drugs with considerable confidence that they will help us and not harm us. But there is no way to make them 100% risk-free. That is why an important "drug scientist" is the consumer, the person who takes the medicine and experiences its effects firsthand.

•   •   •   •

CHAPTER 7

· · · · · · · · · · · · · ·

ON THE
HORIZON

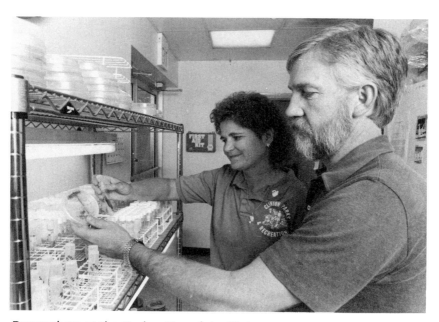

Researchers at the Harbor Branch Institute.

About half the drugs in use today, including aspirin, morphine, and many antibiotics, come from living things. Most of these drugs contain products taken from plants that live on the land. But about 80% of all living things—some 400,000 species of plants and animals—dwell in the ocean. And, according

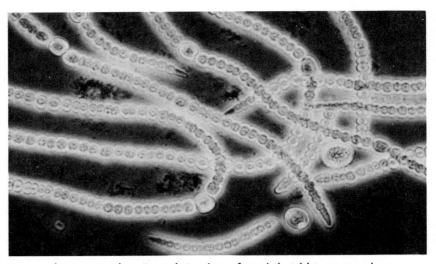

Researchers at Harbor Branch Institute found that blue-green algae (shown here) contains a substance that stimulated the immune system of animals by more than 200%.

to scientists at the Harbor Branch Institute for Oceanographic Research in Fort Pierce, Florida, as many as 10% of the ocean's organisms promise to yield useful drugs.

INNOVATIVE RESEARCH

In 1985 a drug company called SeaPharm teamed up with the Harbor Branch Institute; by 1988 a group of researchers had examined 11,000 ocean creatures and were testing half a dozen new substances as immune-system stimulants, anticancer drugs, or antibiotics. When one substance, derived from a barnaclelike creature called a tunicate, was tested in animals, it acted against melanoma, the most lethal kind of skin cancer. Another substance, derived from blue-green algae, stimulated animals' immune systems by as much as 225% and stimulated immunity of cells in test tubes by 2,000%. Each year SeaPharm sends 2,000 ocean species to the National Cancer Institute, where substances are tested for possible healing properties against 100 different human cancers.

Researchers in California have also made exciting breakthroughs. Joint research carried on by scientists at the Scripps Institute of Oceanography in San Diego and at two state universities—the University of California at Santa Barbara and the

University of California at Santa Cruz—have isolated a compound taken from the *Jasplakina* sponge that seems to fight fungus infections. Other scientists have found the source of a possible new antiarthritis drug in the purple coral sea whip, native to waters off the Florida Keys and the Bahamas. In 1978, small tunicates that live on sponges and corals in the Caribbean Sea were found to contain didemnin-B. Originally tried against viruses, didemnin-B proved effective against cancerous tumors and is currently being tested in human beings in trials sponsored by the National Cancer Institute.

At least one sea creature has already proved invaluable for medicinal purposes. Blood from horseshoe crabs is in worldwide use in hospitals and laboratories as part of a process known as the Limulus amoebocyte lysate test. The test is based on the discovery that when crab blood is exposed to endotoxins (the poisons made by bacteria) it forms a gel. Developed in 1956 by scientist Frederick Bang and his colleague Jack Levin, both of the University of Massachusetts, the Limulus test is a quick and economical way to determine whether a substance contains bacterial contamination.

The reason sea creatures are such rich sources of potential drugs is that they produce many biologically active substances—chemicals that affect living cells. For researchers, the trick is determining which substances are useful. Several clues help scientists narrow down the field. Seemingly defenseless organisms are a good bet. When marine scientists find such creatures, they suspect the presence of unseen substances that might make useful drugs. Consider the sea hare. Because it is a soft mollusk, it has no protective shell; it wards off predators with its repellent taste, which it obtains by eating algae and depositing their toxins (poisons) in its skin. Another likely source of useful substances is brightly colored creatures, which also often produce active substances in their strategy to discourage hungry predators attracted to their brilliant hues.

When modified chemically, poisons often make effective drugs. And substances taken from the sea are among the deadliest of all known poisons. The pufferfish, which lives in several of the world's oceans, contains a high quantity of tetrodotoxin, a particularly lethal poison. Yet the fish is a delicacy in Japan, where highly trained chefs extract all the toxic substance from the puf-

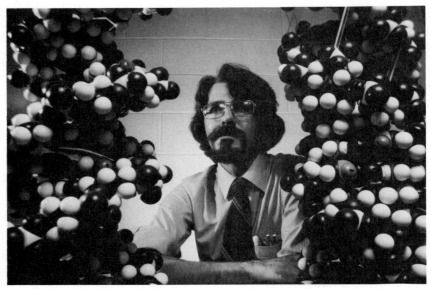

A geneticist with models of molecules. Through genetic engineering, scientists can produce their own supply of substances rather than rely on the limited sources found in nature.

fer, leaving only a tiny bit of poison that causes a tongue-tingling sensation prized by gourmets. Each year, however, several people die from eating the fish. In Haiti, practitioners of Voodooism rub powdered pufferfish toxin, called "zombie powder," into cuts in human skin, causing paralysis and apparent death. Later, when the victim rises, people think he or she has "risen from the dead." When chemically modified, however, tetrodotoxin may produce a topical (applied to skin) painkiller 160,000 times as potent as cocaine.

Genetic Engineering

Extracting substances directly from ocean creatures and other forms of life is difficult, time-consuming, and expensive, and may deplete the original source of a substance. The common mussel, for instance, produces a gooey material that enables it to cling to wet, slippery rocks. This material may prove useful to surgeons and dentists as a glue for fixing damaged or torn tissue. But it takes 3,000 mussels to produce 1 gram of the glue. Thus, instead of raiding the supply of millions of mussels, scientists now produce their own supply of the substance with a technique called genetic engineering. In this process, scientists first locate the gene that tells a mussel's cells to make the glue and then inject the gene into yeast or bacteria cells, which then manufacture mussel glue.

Scientists at the Augouron Institute in La Jolla, California, are using genetic engineering to insert into the bacteria *E. coli* bioluminescent genes, genes that cause certain creatures to glow. The researchers hope to implant bioluminescent genes from *Vibrio fischeri*, a glowing sea bacteria, into other water and some land bacteria, attaching the transplanted genes to distress-signal genes that activate when threatened or damaged by alien matter. A bacteria with a combined glow-distress gene would light up when environmental pollution threatened it—thus flashing a pollution-alert signal to help protect soil or water.

Someday genetically engineered bacteria may also produce vital body chemicals. Indeed, human insulin is currently being prepared for use by diabetics by this process. If a genetically engineered bacteria could also be made to produce insulin inside the human body, diabetes might be controlled much better. For now, such an advance still belongs to the realm of science fiction.

Eventually, research may yield a chemical that will enable diabetics to produce their own supply of insulin rather than have to inject it with a hypodermic needle.

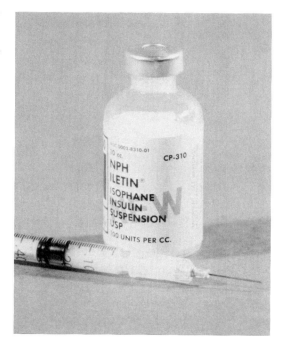

More practically, genetic engineering is already producing new vaccines, including an anticancer vaccine, a birth control vaccine, a vaccine against dengue fever (a mosquito-transmitted disease that causes epidemics in Asia and South America), and a vaccine to prevent malaria. All these vaccines are the products of gene-altered viruses, bacteria, or antibodies (the body's own disease-fighting cells).

The Final Frontier

Outer space, another fertile source of new drugs, has not yet been pursued because space-based laboratories have not yet been built. But such environments will aid scientists greatly because drug making works better in a weightless environment than under normal conditions. Many drugs, for instance, change into solids through crystallization; in a zero-gravity environment large crystals (solids whose molecular structure has a regular geometric form called a lattice) can be made more quickly, easily, and purely. Other drug substances can be mixed only in zero-gravity laboratories.

As space exploration proceeds, drug companies are sure to pursue the opportunities space-based research can provide. Drug research, in fact, is one pursuit expected to reap prompt financial benefits once zero-gravity laboratories become a reality.

Worldly Prizes

Meanwhile, drug companies are already plunging into the contest to develop new substances that will augment sales and profits. Competition can be a healthy spur to research because every company wants to create a unique market. In 1988, for instance, the Chiron Corporation announced it had discovered the virus responsible for a mysterious form of hepatitis, called non-A, non-B hepatitis. Because there has been no way to detect the virus in blood transfusions, the disease is sometimes spread by transfused blood and strikes 150,000 people per year in the United States alone. Twenty percent of its victims develop cirrhosis (liver damage), and some run a high risk of developing liver cancer.

Chiron scientists were reasonably certain which virus caused the disease, but they did not publicize their findings until after they had developed a screening test and applied for patents on their discoveries that would prevent other drug companies from beating them to the punch. The ploy succeeded. Until their patents expire, Chiron will earn an estimated $285 million in annual profits from the new hepatitis test. During the development period, however, Chiron scientists could not be sure some other company was not working on a similar test. The race to be first motivated Chiron researchers to work as hard and fast as possible and resulted in prompt availability of a test that may save thousands of lives per year.

Drug companies profit not only from developing new drugs but also from refining existing treatments. In 1989, the drug company Schering-Plough will probably increase its earnings by 15%, thanks to allergy sufferers who will buy loratadine, an anti-allergy drug—recently developed by the company—that does not induce drowsiness and can be taken only once a day. Similarly, in 1986 Bristol-Meyers introduced Buspar, a tranquilizer that does not interact with alcohol and thus spares consumers dangerous alcohol-drug reactions. Bristol-Meyers may earn $200 million per year on the drug. Cyclosporine, widely used to prevent the body from rejecting tissue and organ transplants, has always

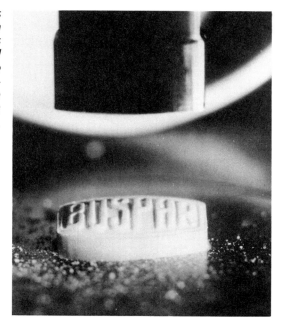

In 1986, Bristol-Meyers introduced Buspar, a tranquilizer that does not interact with alcohol and thus promises to spare consumers dangerous reactions. Here, a tablet of Buspar is being formed.

caused strong and often dangerous side effects, including kidney damage and high blood pressure. In 1988, Oregon Health Sciences University drug researcher William Bennet and his colleague Vickie Kelley at Boston Brigham and Women's Hospital found a new formulation of the drug—by combining it with fish oil—that may reduce kidney damage caused by cyclosporine. Clinical trials are under way to see if fish oil can help organ-transplant patients take cyclosporine without severe kidney damage. If the results are good, a new formulation of cyclosporine with fish oil may reach the market in the early 1990s.

Within Our Grasp

So many substances are under study now that it is impossible to list them all here. Some other examples of potential "wonder drugs" include

- Clomipramine, which blocks a brain chemical called serotonin. Initial reports say the drug may help as many as 5 million people who suffer mental disorders.
- A new use for vitamin A, to block cancers of the mouth.
- A test to detect diabetes very early in the course of the disease, when it is best treated.
- A test to determine whether a cancerous tumor is likely to spread.
- A test to find abnormal cells before they turn into cancerous cells.
- A drug to treat Alzheimer's disease, an illness of the brain that strikes the elderly population in particular.

Pure Research

All these new drug possibilities—and many more—have originated from pure research, the science of finding things out just for the sake of expanding human knowledge. Pure research does not get much funding because it is usually difficult to predict what immediate use the results will have. Yet pure research will probably produce tomorrow's drug miracles.

Scientists John Kao and co-workers at Oak Ridge National Laboratory in Tennessee, for instance, have found that hairy skin absorbs more drug substance than does ordinary skin. They learned this by testing drugs on bald mice. What could be more useless, one might ask, than studying bald mice? Yet Kao's work may provide more effective and less painful methods for administering drugs and even allow some new drugs to work when they otherwise might not. Kao's studies may also help prevent some diseases, such as cancers, that are caused by pollution absorbed through the skin.

Drugs have been used to combat disease for thousands of years, but over the past century progress in discovering and using them has led to medical miracles: drugs that are safer, more powerful, and more available than ever before. A century ago it was common for people to die of infected teeth, for example, because there was no treatment that kept an infection from spreading to the rest of the body. Today antibiotics cure such infections with relative ease, and death from them is almost unheard of.

A century from now fearsome diseases, even cancer, may be cured as easily as minor infections are cured today. Meanwhile, many diseases remain to challenge drug researchers. We all can

Researchers at Oak Ridge National Laboratory tested drugs on these bald mice. The results may help provide more effective and less painful ways of administering drugs to humans.

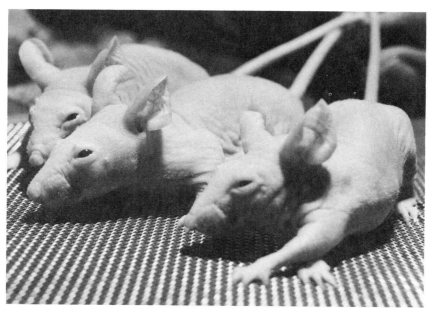

take comfort, however, in this fact: More and better drugs to promote health and fight disease are available now than at any time in history. Progress is being made—and more is certain to come—in preventing and curing ills that diminish our health and happiness.

•   •   •   •

•   •   •   •   •   •   •   •

APPENDIX 1:
A CHECKLIST OF
COMMON PRESCRIPTION AND
OTC DRUGS

The following list is a guide to commonly used remedies. Each entry describes the drug's effects, side effects, safety, and—if called for—its interactions with foods or other drugs.

Acetaminophen: an OTC pain-relief drug available under many brand names, including Tylenol, Datril, and Liquiprin. Its effects and side effects are similar to those of aspirin (see **Aspirin**, below) except that acetaminophen has no anti-inflammatory action and so it is not useful as an arthritis treatment. Overdosage of acetaminophen is dangerous because the drug can endanger the liver.

Aspirin: the common name for acetylsalicylic acid, an OTC pain-relief drug sold under many brand names, including Bayer Aspirin, St. Joseph's Aspirin, Bufferin, and Empirin. It is used to treat pain, fever, and inflammation. Its side effects may include stomach pain, diarrhea, lowered blood clotting and increased bleeding, ringing in the ears, and allergic reactions. Aspirin should be used cautiously by allergy sufferers, people suffering from alcohol hangover, bleeding conditions, anemia, or stomach ulcers, or by anyone who is pregnant or soon to have surgery. It should not be taken during or after a flulike illness by people under 16 years old: Such use has been linked to Reye's syndrome, a fatal complication of viral illnesses. Aspirin interacts with many other drugs; hence, anyone taking a prescription drug should consult with a physician before taking aspirin.

Benzoyl peroxide: the active drug ingredient in many OTC antiacne products, including Clearasil, Oxy-5, Oxy-10, and Oxy Wash. It kills bacteria, removes excess oil, and prevents oil plugs from clogging skin pores. Its side effects may include redness and irritation. Products containing benzoyl peroxide should be used carefully and over a period of several months in order to achieve their full effects. The user should start with a low-strength product and rinse it off after 15 minutes so that the skin can adjust to the irritation caused by the substance—the neck is a particularly sensitive area. Benzoyl peroxide products can make people susceptible to sunburn and therefore should not be used while sunbathing. Some people may find that the drug causes skin peeling. It can also stain hair and clothes. People being treated for acne should not use benzoyl peroxide products without first consulting their physician: Combining the drug with prescription antiacne medications may injure skin.

Chlorpropamide: manufactured by Pfizer Laboratories Divisions under the brand name Diabinese. Diabinese is used to treat some forms of diabetes. Its side effects may include diarrhea, dizziness, fatigue, headache, rash, vomiting, and weakness. It is not effective in children under age 12, and it should not be used by people with severe infections, severe injuries, or who are about to have surgery. Because Diabinese interacts with many other drugs, people taking it should make sure their doctor is aware of any other drugs they are taking. Diabinese should not be combined with alcohol. It is available only by prescription.

Diazepam: a tranquilizer manufactured by Roche Products Inc. under the brand name Valium. Valium is used to treat anxiety, muscle spasms, and symptoms of withdrawal from alcohol addiction. Its side effects may include confusion, constipation, depression, drowsiness, headache, nausea, and other major side effects. It should not be used by people afflicted with certain types of glaucoma, by pregnant women, or by people with suicidal tendencies. Valium interacts with other sedatives and with alcohol and should not be combined with them. Valium is addictive and is available only by prescription.

Diphenhydramine hydrochloride: manufactured by Parke-Davis under the brand name Benadryl. An antiallergy drug, Benadryl is used for treatment of itching and swelling. It may also be used against nausea caused by motion sickness. Side effects may include blurred vision, confusion, constipation, drowsiness, headache, nervousness, and palpitations (rapid heartbeat). It should not be used by people with asthma, glaucoma (an eye disease), stomach ulcers, liver disease, kidney disease, or during pregnancy. It should not be combined with alcohol. Benadryl is available both by prescription and as an OTC product.

Diphenoxylate hydrochloride and **atropine sulfate:** manufactured by Searle & Co. under the brand name Lomotil. Lomotil is used to relieve diarrhea. Its side effects may include abdominal pain, itching, rash, dizziness, drowsiness, fever, headache, breathing difficulties, and swollen gums. Lomotil should not be combined with alcohol, and people using it should drink eight or nine glasses of water per day. The drug should not be used for more than five days except on a doctor's orders. Lomotil is available only by prescription.

Erythromycin: an antibiotic drug whose brand names include E-Mycin and Ilosone. Erythromycin is used to treat a wide variety of bacterial infections. Its side effects may include abdominal cramps, diarrhea, fatigue, fever, and vomiting. It should not be taken during the first three months of pregnancy. Erythromycin should be taken for a full ten days even if symptoms disappear. It is available only by prescription.

Gamma benzene hexachloride: also caled lindane, manufactured by Reed & Carnrick under the brand name Kwell. Kwell is a lotion or shampoo used to kill head lice, crab lice, and other skin parasites. Its side effects can be toxic, and therefore it should be applied with great caution; less serious side effects may include rash and skin irritation. Kwell should never be swallowed: It is poisonous when taken internally. Kwell is available only by prescription.

Hexachlorophene: a drug that kills bacteria on the skin, used in an OTC skin soap manufactured by Winthrop Laboratories under the brand name pHisoHex. Its side effects may include skin irritation. Hexachlorophene should not be used on open wounds, on burns, in the eyes, or on infants. It must be rinsed off after use. If used incorrectly, hexachlorophene may be absorbed into the body and cause harm to the brain and nervous system.

Hydrocortisone: a steroid hormone (a substance similar to those produced naturally by some body glands) used to reduce inflammation and itching of poison ivy and other skin irritations. It is available in 5% strengths in OTC skin ointments such as Cortaid and Aristocort. It should never be used on or in the eyes or by anyone with an infection. If skin irritations do not clear up after use of 5% hydrocortisone, the sufferer should see a physician.

Ibuprofen: an OTC pain reliever available under several brand names, including Advil and Nuprin. Ibuprofen treats pain and inflammation arising from many causes, including headaches, menstrual cramps, and arthritis. Unlike aspirin, it does not reduce fever. Its side effects may include heartburn, nausea, nervousness, increased bleeding tendency, rash, and other side effects. People allergic to aspirin should consult a physician before taking ibuprofen products, which can interact with other drugs. Potential users should consult a doctor.

Insulin: used to treat diabetes, a disease that disables the digestive system from using sugar properly. Its major side effect is low blood sugar, which can cause dizziness, fainting, and coma. Because insulin interacts with other drugs, it should not be taken in conjunction with any other drug or remedy unless a doctor approves. Proper dosage of insulin is crucial to its safe use; thus people using the drug should check carefully that the dose is the correct one. Insulin is available only by prescription.

Meperidine hydrochloride: manufactured by Winthrop Laboratories under the brand name Demerol. Demerol is a controlled narcotic used for the relief of severe pain. Side effects may include nausea, vomiting, fainting, sweating, breathing problems, and low blood pressure. Demerol should not be used by people with head injuries, breathing problems, or epilepsy unless a doctor provides careful supervision. The drug should not be combined with alcohol. Demerol is addictive and is available only by prescription.

Miconazole: a combination antifungus and antibacterial drug, available OTC under the brand name Micatin. Micatin is an athlete's foot remedy that also relieves itching. Like all such medications, it must be used faithfully and regularly in combination with good foot hygiene. Improvement may not appear for three weeks; any longer, however, and the user should consult a doctor.

Nystatin: manufactured by E. R. Squibb & Sons, Inc. under the brand name Mycostatin. Mycostatin is used for the treatment of fungus infections, especially of the feet, mouth, and vagina. Its side effects may include itching, rash, diarrhea, and vomiting. It should not be used during the first three months of pregnancy. Mycostatin should be used according to the instructions supplied with it and is available only by prescription.

Oral contraceptives: drugs women take by mouth to prevent unwanted pregnancy or to regulate the menstrual cycle. Minor side effects may include nausea, dizziness, and abdominal cramps. Major side effects may include fluid retention, high blood pressure, and stroke. To reduce the risks of major side effects, oral contraceptives should be used cautiously, if at all, by women over 35, smokers, and women afflicted with high blood pressure or heart disease. They should not be taken by women with eye ailments, bleeding abnormalities, diabetes, gall bladder disease, or migraine headaches. Because they interfere with other drugs, women using oral contraceptives should make sure their doctor is aware of any other drugs they are taking. Oral contraceptives must be taken regularly according to instructions. Missing even one dose may allow pregnancy to occur. Oral contraceptives are available only by prescription and should be taken only under the supervision of a physician.

Penicillin: an antibiotic available under several brand names, including Pentids (manufactured by E. R. Squibb & Sons, Inc.). Potassium phenoxymethyl penicillin, another penicillin form, is available under the brand name Pen-Vee K, manufactured by Wyeth Laboratories, as well as under other brand names. Penicillin treats a wide variety of bacterial infections. It works best when taken on an empty stomach. Its side effects may include diarrhea, nausea, rash, and vomiting. The drug should be used with extreme care by people who have asthma or other allergies. It should not be used by people allergic to penicillin or to ampicillin. It interacts with chloramphenicol, erythromycin, tetracycline, and with foods high in acid (such as orange juice) when the drug is taken orally. Diabetics using penicillin should use Clinistix or Tes-Tape to test their urine because Clinitest may show a false high sugar reading in the presence of penicillin. Penicillin is available only by prescription.

Phenylephrine: a decongestant drug (used against "stuffy nose") found in OTC products, including Sinarest and Neo-Synephrine. Its side effects may include nervousness, rapid heartbeat, shakiness, and rebound, wherein congestion worsens once the drug wears off. Phenylephrine is effective when used in topical products such as nose sprays, but in oral remedies it is not very effective because little is absorbed through the intestinal tract. Phenylephrine interacts with other drugs; hence, potential users should consult a doctor.

Phenytoin sodium and **diphenylhydantoin:** manufactured by Parke-Davis under the brand name Dilantin. Dilantin is used to control epilepsy and other seizure disorders. Its side effects may include constipation, gum swelling, headache, drowsiness, rash, vomiting, dizziness, and slurred speech. It should not be taken during the first three months of pregnancy or by people with liver or kidney disease. Because Dilantin interacts with many drugs, people taking it should make sure their physician is aware of any other drugs they are taking. Dilantin should not be combined with alcohol. People should discontinue their use of Dilantin gradually, so that seizures do not result. Good dental care is also important: The drug can cause the gums to enlarge. Dilantin is available only by prescription.

Prednisone: a steroid hormone (a substance similar to that produced by the body's glands) available under many brand names, including Oracort and Lisacort. It is used to treat many kinds of inflammation, including severe allergies, asthma, and arthritis and is combined with other drugs to keep the body from rejecting transplanted organ tissue. Its side effects may include headache, dizziness, sweating, fluid retention, eye ailments, stomach ulcers, high blood pressure, and other major side effects. It should not be used by people with infections, ulcers, tuberculosis, or during pregnancy. Prednisone and other steroids interact with many drugs and should be taken strictly according to a physician's orders. It can cause potassium loss, which may be remedied by a change in diet or by potassium supplements. Weight and blood pressure should be monitored regularly in people taking the drug, which is available only by prescription.

Selenium sulfide: used in a shampoo manufactured by Abbott Laboratories under the brand name Selsun for treatment of dandruff and other skin diseases of the scalp. Its side effects may include hair color change, scalp dryness, and skin irritation. It should not be used if the scalp is inflamed. The drug is harmful when swallowed and should only be applied to the scalp. Selsun is available only by prescription. A less powerful form of selenium sulfide is available in the OTC shampoo Selsun Blue.

Sulfisoxazole and **penazopyridine hydrochloride:** manufactured by Roche Products, Inc. under the brand name Gantrisin. Gantrisin, which is composed of an antibiotic (sulfisoxazole) and a pain reliever (penazopyridine hydrochloride), is used to treat bacterial infections of the urinary tract. Its side effects may include diarrhea, headache, nausea, vomiting, fluid retention, itching, rash, ringing in the ears, and sore throat. Gantrisin should not be taken during the first three months of pregnancy and should be used cautiously by people with asthma or other allergies, conditions it can worsen. Because Gantrisin interacts with many other drugs, people who take it, especially diabetics, should inform their physician of any other drugs they are taking. Gantrisin is available only by prescription.

Tetracycline: an antibiotic available under many brand names, including Achromycin and Panmycin. It is used for the treatment of a wide variety of infections, including severe acne. Its side effects may include diarrhea, rash, itching, sore throat, blood disorders, and increased sensitivity to sunlight; persons taking tetracycline should avoid prolonged exposure to the sun because they may burn more rapidly and severely than under ordinary circumstances. It should not be used in the first three months of pregnancy or by children under age nine except under the careful supervision of a doctor. Tetracycline interacts with many other drugs and with dairy products and some antacids, thus people using tetracycline should notify their physician of any other drugs they are taking. Tetracycline should be ingested on an empty stomach and should be taken for a full ten days even if symptoms disappear. The drug is available only by prescription.

Vitamins and minerals: substances the body requires in very tiny amounts in order to perform its functions properly. People who eat a balanced diet do not need vitamin supplements except under conditions, such as prolonged fever, broken bones, major infections, and major surgery, that lead to physical stress. Nursing mothers, heavy drinkers, and people with diseases that impair vitamin absorption should have vitamin supplements prescribed by a doctor. Other people whose diets do not supply their vitamin needs require better diets, not vitamin pills. Vitamins are not harmless; overdose may cause illness or death. Some vitamins are stored by the body and can cause severe harm if taken over a long period of time. Regular use of a "multiple vitamin" is unlikely, however, to cause harm, although the benefits yielded by multiple vitamins, if any, are still under debate.

APPENDIX 2:
WHEN NOT TO TREAT
WITH OTC DRUGS

Some symptoms should not be treated with OTC remedies because they may mask symptoms without treating the underlying cause. If you have any of the symptoms listed below, do not try to remedy them yourself. Instead, see your physician.

ACNE: See a doctor if the things you do to relieve acne do not work or make outbreaks worse, or you have hard lumps under your skin, or you have large patches of acne, or if you are more than 20 years old.

ALLERGIES (HAY FEVER): See a doctor if you get no relief from over-the-counter drugs, if your nasal mucus is yellow or green, if you get pain above your teeth, on the sides of your nose, or around your eyes, or if you develop an earache.

ATHLETE'S FOOT: See a doctor if you have diabetes, if your toenails are involved, if your skin has white or soggy patches, if your foot oozes, gets red, or begins to swell.

COLD SORES: See a doctor if a cold sore lasts more than a week or if it oozes yellow material.

CONSTIPATION: See a doctor if you have constipation for more than two weeks, if you have pain when trying to pass stools, if you have blood in your stools, or if you have pain, bloating, weight loss, fever, or upset stomach.

COUGHS AND COLDS: See a doctor if your cold lasts longer than a week; if sore throat with a cold lasts longer than two days; if your nose or throat mucus is yellow or green; if you get a bad stiff neck, a severe headache, pain above your teeth, on the side of your nose, or around your eyes; or if you develop an earache.

DANDRUFF: See a doctor if you have red or scaly scalp areas, if your dandruff does not improve after shampooing with OTC dandruff soap, or if you have severe itching.

DIARRHEA: See a doctor if you are pregnant, if your stomach is sore to touch, if you have a fever, if you lose more than a couple of pounds, if your diarrhea lasts more than two days, or if your stools are bloody or black.

EXCESS WEIGHT: There are no over-the-counter drugs that are safe or effective for inducing weight loss.

EYE AND EAR PROBLEMS: See a doctor for any eye injury, eye pain, blurred vision, continuous tearing, for a "black eye," for a foreign object in the eye, or for continuing dryness of the eye. See a doctor if you have ear pain, fluid coming from the ear, or hearing loss.

FEVER: See a doctor if your fever goes over 103°F or 39.5°C, if fever lasts more than three days, if aspirin or acetaminophen does not reduce fever, if you have pain when you pass urine, or if you have difficulty breathing.

HEADACHE: See a doctor if you have severe pain, stiff neck, fever with headache, vision changes, weakness, loss of feeling in any body part, or confusion, drowsiness, or personality changes.

HEMORRHOIDS: See a doctor for treatment of hemorrhoids.

INSOMNIA: See your doctor if you cannot sleep well for more than two weeks, if you have weight loss, weight gain, anxiety, if you feel depressed and wake up too early each morning, or if your sleep problems are due to other symptoms such as pain or shortness of breath.

JOINT AND MUSCLE PAIN: See a doctor if you have intense or sudden pain, if pain is accompanied by fever, if you cannot move a body part, if you have numbness or tingling, or if you have arthritis.

MENSTRUAL CRAMPS: See a doctor if your menstrual pattern or the appearance of your menses changes, you have noticeable swelling, your cramps cause pain that limits your normal activities, or you have unusual fatigue or any shortness of breath.

NERVOUSNESS: There are no over-the-counter drugs that are safe or effective for nervousness. See your doctor if your nervousness interferes with your normal activities or causes you more discomfort than you think is normal.

NUTRITION: See your doctor if you have any digestive disease, if you often feel tired, if you are pale, or if you feel a general lack of energy.

POISON IVY: See a doctor if your itching is severe, if your poison ivy rash covers a large area, if your rash is near your eyes, if large blisters develop, if the rash exudes yellow liquid, if you develop swelling, or if fever develops.

SKIN INFECTIONS: Infected skin should always be treated by a physician. See a doctor if you show signs of skin infection including redness, oozing of yellow or green material, warmth or swelling at the infected place, a wound that heals slowly or not at all, or if you have diabetes.

SORE THROAT: See a doctor if a sore throat lasts more than a week, if you have chills or high fever, if you have swollen glands, difficulty breathing, or difficulty swallowing liquids.

VOMITING: See a doctor if your vomiting lasts more than three days or is severe, if you cannot keep fluids down, if you vomit blood or material that looks like coffee grounds, if you have pain or fever, or if your stomach swells.

APPENDIX 3:
FOR MORE INFORMATION

GENERAL INFORMATION

The following organizations can provide information regarding prescription and over-the-counter drugs.

National Organization for Rare Disorders
(203) 746-6518
For information on orphan drugs or other treatment of rare diseases.

U.S. Food and Drug Administration
5600 Fishers Lane
Rockville, MD 20857
For information on laws regulating drugs, new drug testing and development, drug safety and effectiveness.

PHARMACEUTICAL ASSOCIATIONS

The following pharmaceutical associations can provide information on drug research, the use of drugs, and pharmaceutical practices.

Academy of Pharmacy Practice (APP)
c/o American Pharmaceutical Association
2215 Constitution Avenue NW
Washington, DC 20037
(202) 628-4410

Alliance for the Prudent Use of Antibiotics
PO Box 1372
Boston, MA 02117
(617) 956-6765

American Institute of the History of Pharmacy
Pharmacy Building
425 North Chater Street
Madison, WI 53706
(608) 262-5378

American Pharmaceutical Association
2215 Constitution Avenue NW
Washington, DC 20037
(202) 628-4410

American Society for Pharmacology and Experimental Therapeutics
9650 Rockville Pike
Bethesda, MD 20814
(301) 530-7060

Drug Information Association
PO Box 133
Maple Glen, PA 19002
(215) 628-2288

National Association of Boards of Pharmacy
1300 Higgins Road, Suite 103
Park Ridge, IL 60068
(312) 698-6227

National Council on Patient
Information and Education
1625 I Street NW, Suite 1010
Washington, DC 20006
(202) 466-6711

National Pharmaceutical
Association
c/o College of Pharmacy &
Pharmacal Sciences
Howard University
Washington, DC 20059
(202) 328-9229

PHARMACEUTICAL EDUCATION

*The following organizations provide
information about pharmacy education and careers.*

American Association of Colleges of
Pharmacy
1426 Prince Street
Alexandria, VA 22314
(703) 739-2330

American Council on
Pharmaceutical Education
311 West Superior Street, Suite 512
Chicago, IL 60610

National Association of Boards of
Pharmacy
One East Wacker Drive, Suite 2210
Chicago, IL 60601

DRUG EDUCATION

*The following organizations provide
information to those who want to
educate students and adults about
drug use and abuse.*

PRIDE/National Parents Resource
Institute for Drug Education
(800) 241-7946

Project Inform
(800) 822-7422

STATE AND LOCAL DRUG ABUSE TREATMENT CENTERS

*The following list provides the
names and addresses of some drug
abuse treatment programs that provide information and assistance to
adolescents around the country.*

ALABAMA

Alternatives Inc.
Drug Abuse Treatment Unit
PO Box 341
Wetumpka, AL 36092
(205) 567-7083

ARIZONA

Rehab of Mesa Inc.
Alcoholism/Drug Abuse Treatment
Units
PO Drawer G
Mesa, AZ 85201
(602) 969-4024

CALIFORNIA

Awareness Program
Drug Abuse Treatment Center
1153 Oak Street
San Francisco, CA 94115
(415) 431-9000

CONNECTICUT

Regional Network Program
171 Golden Hill Street
Bridgeport, CT 06604
(203) 333-4105

FLORIDA

Turnabout
2531 West Tharpe Street
PO Box 13488
Tallahassee, FL 32303
(904) 385-5179

PRESCRIPTION AND OVER-THE-COUNTER DRUGS

GEORGIA

Clayton Outpatient Program
Drug Abuse Treatment Unit
6315 Don Hastings Drive
Flint River Center
Riverdale, GA 30274
(404) 991-0111

HAWAII

Awareness House Inc.
Alcoholism/Drug Abuse Treatment
Unit
305 Wailuku Drive
Hilo, HI 96720
(808) 961-4771

ILLINOIS

Northwest Youth Outreach Drug
Abuse Treatment
Alcoholism/Drug Abuse Treatment
Unit
6417 West Irving Park Road
Chicago, IL 60634
(312) 777-7112

INDIANA

Aquarius House
Alcoholism/Drug Abuse Treatment
413 S. Liberty
Muncie, IN 46015
(317) 282-2257

LOUISIANA

Education and Treatment Council
Inc.
Alcoholism/Drug Abuse Treatment
Unit
1146 Hodges
Lake Charles, LA 70601
(318) 433-1062

MAINE

Saco Unit
Alcoholism/Drug Abuse Treatment
Unit
265 North Street
Saco, ME 04072
(207) 282-7504

MARYLAND

Youth Services Program
Harbel Drug Abuse
5807 Harford Road
Baltimore, MD 21214
(301) 444-2100

MASSACHUSETTS

Project Concern
Drug Abuse Treatment Unit
1000 Harvard Street
Boston, MA 02126
(617) 298-0106

MICHIGAN

The Center For Human
Resources
1113 Military Street
Port Huron, MI 48060
(313) 985-5168

MINNESOTA

Warren Eustis House
720 O'Neill Drive
Eagan, MN 55121
(612) 452-6908

NEVADA

Bridge Counseling Associates
Alcoholism/Drug Abuse Treatment
Unit
1785 East Sahara, Suite 130
Las Vegas, NV 89104
(702) 734-6070

NEW HAMPSHIRE

Office of Youth Services
36 Lowell Street
Manchester, NH 03101
(603) 624-6470

NEW JERSEY

Woodbridge Action for Youth
Drug Abuse Treatment Unit
73 Green Street
Woodbridge, NJ 07095
(201) 634-7910

NEW MEXICO

Behavioral Health Services of
    Acoma
Substance Abuse Prevention
    Program
PO Box 328
Pueblo of Acoma, NM 87034
(505) 552-6663

NEW YORK

Phase Piggy Back Inc.
Youth Intervention and
    Development
Drug Abuse Treatment Unit
458 West 145th Street
New York, NY 10031
(212) 234-1660

Threshold
115 S. Clinton Avenue
Rochester, NY 14604
(716) 454-7530

OHIO

Choices
Westside CMHC
8711 Dennison Avenue
Cleveland, OH 44102
(216) 631-8686

PENNSYLVANIA

Philadelphia Psychiatric Center
Wurzel Clinic
Ford Road and Monument Avenues
Philadelphia, PA 19131
(215) 581-3757

RHODE ISLAND

Caritas House Inc.
Drug Abuse Treatment Unit
166 Pawtucket Avenue
Pawtucket, RI 02860
(401) 722-4644

TEXAS

United Medical Centers
610 South Monroe
Eagle Pass, TX 78852
(512) 425-7080

VIRGINIA

Bacon Street Inc.
Drug Abuse Treatment Unit
105 Bacon Avenue
Williamsburg, VA 23185
(804) 253-0111

WASHINGTON

Youth Eastside Services
Drug Abuse Treatment Unit
257 100th Avenue NE
Bellevue, WA 98004
(206) 454-5502

WEST VIRGINIA

Western District Guidance Center
Alcoholism/Drug Abuse Treatment
    Unit
2121 Seventh Street
Parkersburg, WV 26101
(304) 485-1721

WISCONSIN

The Recovery Center
County Highway Z
Parkland East Building Box 58A
Wentworth, WI 54894
(715) 398-7646

*TOLL-FREE HOT LINES AND
HELP LINES*

(800) 662-HELP
Operated by the National Institute
    of Drug Abuse

(800) 554-KIDS
Operated by the National
    Federation of Parents for Drug-
    Free Youth. Open 9:00 A.M. to
    5:00 P.M. Eastern Standard time.
    Answers questions and sends
    information to parents who call
    about their youngster's drug
    problems. Not a crisis line.
    Provides no counseling.

Brattleboro Retreat
VT (800) 622-4492
CT, MA, ME, NH, NJ, NY (within area codes: 212, 315, 516, 518, 607, 914), RI (800) 451-4203
All other states including NY area codes not listed above: (800) 622-4492
Receives adult and adolescent in-patients.

Naples Research and Counseling Center
FL (800) 722-0100
Rest of U.S. (800) 282-3508
Information on alcohol, food, and drug addiction; specializes in in-patient treatment.

FURTHER READING

American Association of Retired Persons. *The AARP Pharmacy Service Prescription Drug Handbook*. Des Plaines, IL: Scott, Foresman, 1984.

American Society of Hospital Pharmacists. *Consumer Drug Digest*. New York: Facts on File, 1982.

Check, William. *Drugs of the Future*. New York: Chelsea House, 1987.

Clayman, Charles B., ed. *The American Medical Association Guide to Prescription and Over-the-Counter Drugs*. New York: Random House, 1988.

Edwards, Gabrielle I. *Coping with Drug Abuse*. Rev. ed. New York: Rosen, 1988.

Food and Drug Administration. *New Drug Development in the United States*. Washington, DC: Food and Drug Administration, 1988.

Gilman, A. Z., and L. S. Goodman, eds. *The Pharmacological Basis for Therapeutics*. 7th ed. New York: Macmillan, 1985.

Goth, Andres, ed. *Medical Pharmacology*. St. Louis, MO: Mosby, 1985.

Grogan, F. J. *The Pharmacist's Prescription*. New York: Rawson, 1972.

Henningfield, Jack E., and Nancy Almand Ator. *Barbiturates*. New York: Chelsea House, 1986.

Lukas, Scott E. *Amphetamines*. New York: Chelsea House, 1985.

Margolin, S., and R. M. Schmidt, eds. *Harper's Handbook of Therapeutic Pharmacy*. New York: Harper & Row, 1981.

Medical Economics Company. *Physicians' Desk Reference*. 43rd ed. Oradell, NJ: Medical Economics Company, 1989.

Medical Economics Company. *Physicians' Desk Reference for Nonprescription Drugs*. 9th ed. Oradell, NJ: Medical Economics Company, 1988.

Nassif, Janet Zhum. *Handbook of Health Careers*. New York: Human Sciences Press, 1980.

Rodman, Morton J., and Amy M. Karch, eds. *Pharmacology and Drug Therapy in Nursing*. Philadelphia: Lippincott, 1985.

Sandberg, Paul, and Richard M. T. Krema. *Over-the-Counter Drugs*. New York: Chelsea House, 1986.

Stern, Edward L. *Prescription Drugs and Their Side Effects*. New York: Perigee, 1983.

The United States Department of Health and Human Services. *New Drug Development in the United States*. FDA Pub. #88-3168. Rockville, MD, 1988.

The United States Department of Health and Human Services. *The OTC Drug Review*. FDA Pub. 1087. Rockville, MD, 1988.

United States Pharmacopeia Convention. *USP DI: United States Pharmacopeia Dispensing Information*. 2 vols. 8th ed. Rockville, MD: United States Pharmacopeia Convention, 1988.

Winger, Gail. *Valium*. New York: Chelsea House, 1986.

Wolfe, Sidney. *Pills That Don't Work*. New York: Farrar, Straus & Giroux, 1981.

Zimmerman, David R., *The Essential Guide to Nonprescription Drugs*. New York: Harper & Row, 1983.

GLOSSARY

addiction a condition caused by repeated drug use, characterized by a compulsive urge to continue using a certain drug, a tendency to increase dosage, and/or psychological dependence

amphetamine any one of a number of drugs that act to stimulate parts of the central nervous system

ampule a glass container in which drugs can be kept sterile; each ampule usually holds one dose of a specific medication

analgesic a drug that relieves pain

anatomy the study of the structure of the body

antihistamine any one of various compounds used to combat allergic reactions, cold symptoms, and motion sickness

antibiotic a substance produced by or derived from a microorganism and able, when placed in a solution, to inhibit or kill another microorganism; used to combat infection caused by microorganisms and bacteria

anti-inflammatory a drug that relieves redness, swelling, itching, and pain

antiseptic any of a number of substances used to prevent infection during surgery or to disinfect a wound

bacteria unicellular organisms that lack a distinct nuclear membrane; some bacteria cause diseases that can be treated with antibiotics such as penicillin

barbiturate any one of a number of drugs that cause depression of the central nervous system; generally used to reduce anxiety or to induce euphoria

bioequivalent having the same effect and strength on the body as another drug of equal dosage

bronchodilator a drug that relaxes bronchial muscle

capsule drug container made of gelatin; the container dissolves in the stomach, releasing the drug

cardiac having to do with the heart

chaulmoogra oil prescribed treatment for leprosy

clinical trial controlled tests of a drug or other treatment

contraceptive any method, such as use of contraceptive drugs, that prevents pregnancy

contraindication situation or condition indicating that a certain drug ought not to be used

crude drug medication that consists of fresh or dried plant or animal material

diuretic a substance, especially a drug, that helps the body excrete urine

elixir a solution of a drug in alcohol

enkephalin a substance in the brain that acts as the body's own analgesic

enzyme a substance produced by living cells that, although not participating in a given chemical reaction, promotes its speed

gel a solution of a drug in a thick liquid with the consistency of paste

general anesthetic a drug that induces unconsciousness to reduce pain during surgery

generic drug a drug manufactured and sold by drug companies other than the company that first developed and patented it; generics are usually less expensive than the brand-name drug

genetic engineering method of altering the inherited instruction codes within a cell

glomeruli membranes in the kidneys that excrete drugs and by-products of drug-laden blood

hemoglobin a substance in red blood cells that can bind with oxygen and carry it to cells and also carry carbon dioxide away from them

hormone a substance carried in the bloodstream that regulates many bodily processes, modifying both their function and the structure of their cells

immune system the body's defense system against foreign substances

inscription on a prescription, the list of ingredients and prescribed usage amount for the drug

insulin a protein hormone produced in the pancreas and important to the regulation of the blood-sugar level; lack of this hormone may lead to diabetes, a condition in which an excessive amount of sugar is present in the blood and urine because the body is not able to metabolize; diabetes may be treated by injections of insulin

ipecac a crude drug made from the dried, powdered root of the ipecacuanha plant; used to induce vomiting and often administered to people who have swallowed something poisonous

kushta a plant used in ancient Eastern cultures to help people with eye trouble

legend drug a drug restricted by the FDA to use and sale by prescription only

local anesthetic a drug that relieves pain in one area without causing unconsciousness

narcotic originally a group of drugs derived from opium, a product of the poppy plant *Papaver somniferum*, that produce effects similar to those of morphine; often used to refer to any substance that sedates, has a depressant effect, and may cause dependence

orphan drug a drug used so rarely that it is unprofitable to manufacture and therefore is not marketed or developed

over-the-counter drug medication legally obtainable without a doctor's prescription

pathophysiology the study of the effect of diseases on the body

pharmacist a person licensed to dispense prescription drugs

physiology the study of the way the body works

placebo a drug with no active chemical ingredient that nonetheless may relieve symptoms because the patient believes it will

prescription a physician's written order for a drug

rauwolfia a sedative used in ancient Eastern cultures to lower blood pressure

recipere Latin for "take thou;" the superscription, or Rx, that appears on a prescription form

ribosome a protein-making structure in cells

signature the prescription directions printed on the label of the drug container

solution a liquid in which a drug has been dissolved

soma an intoxicating plant juice used in ancient Indian cultures as a drink of immortality and an offering to the gods

subscription on a prescription form, the direction from the doctor for compounding the drug

suppository a drug embedded in a waxy or fat-containing material that liquefies after insertion into a body orifice

suspension a drug mixed into a liquid but not dissolved in it

syrup a drug dissolved in a sugar-containing liquid

tablet a drug dosage made by compressing the drug and an inert material such as starch or sugar into a hard mass. Drugs that irritate the stomach may be coated with a substance that will not dissolve until the pill passes through the stomach and enters the intestine

tetrahydrocannabinol (THC) the active ingredient in marijuana; administered as a drug it can ease the symptoms of glaucoma and also the pain caused by chemotherapy

tetrodotoxin a powerful poison produced by the puffer fish

thymine substance necessary for cells to produce DNA

tincture a concentrated solution of a drug in alcohol

toxicology the study of unwanted or dangerous effects of substances

tranquilizer a drug that relieves anxiety by inducing relaxing and calming effects

vaccine an injection of a usually weakened or dead virus into the bloodstream to produce immunity to the same virus in a person or animal

vitamins organic substances, present naturally in food, that are required (in minute amounts) for healthy growth and development. Insufficient amounts of any of the necessary vitamins can result in specific vitamin-deficiency diseases.

INDEX

PICTURE CREDITS

Elinor S. Beckwith/Taurus Photos: pp. 52, 75; The Bettmann Archive: pp. 15, 16, 18, 19, 21, 23, 48; Bristol-Meyers: p. 83; Laimute Druskis/Taurus Photos: p. 61; Charles Marden Fitch/Taurus Photos: 17, 47; Harber Branch Institute: pp. 67, 77; Pam Hasegawa/Taurus Photos: p. 13; Ellis Herwig/ Taurus Photos: p. 81; Eric Kroll/Taurus Photos: pp. 39, 50; Phiz Mezey/ Taurus Photos: p. 54; Cliff Moore/Taurus Photos: p. 26; Oak Ridge National Laboratory: p. 85; Alfred Pasieka/Taurus Photos: cover; Pfizer Inc.: pp. 25, 27, 29, 40, 51, 72; David M. Phillips/Taurus Photos: p. 28; Martin M. Rotker/ Taurus Photos: pp. 33, 46, 57, 61, 68, 81; S.L.O.T.S./Taurus Photos: p. 64; James Somers/Taurus Photos: p. 78; Taurus Photos: p. 49; Victor & Victor Consultants: p. 65; Richard Wood/Taurus Photos: pp. 31, 45, 53, 70; Original illustrations by Nisa Rauschenberg: pp. 36, 37

Mary Kittredge, a former associate editor of the medical journal *Respiratory Care*, is now a free-lance writer of nonfiction and fiction. She is the author of *Organ Transplants* and *The Respiratory System* in the Chelsea House ENCYCLOPEDIA OF HEALTH. Her writing awards include the Ruell Crompton Tuttle Essay Prize and the Mystery Writers of America Robert L. Fish Award for best first short-mystery fiction of 1986. Ms. Kittredge received a B.A. from Trinity College in Hartford, Connecticut, and studied at the University of California Medical Center, San Francisco. Certified as a respiratory-care technician by the American Association for Respiratory Therapy, she has been a member of the respiratory-care staff at Yale-New Haven Hospital and Medical Center since 1972.

Dale C. Garell, M.D., is medical director of California Childrens Services, Department of Health Services, County of Los Angeles. He is also clinical professor in the Department of Pediatrics and Family Medicine at the University of Southern California School of Medicine and Visiting associate clinical professor of maternal and child health at the University of Hawaii School of Public Health. From 1963 to 1974, he was medical director of the Division of Adolescent Medicine at Children's Hospital in Los Angeles. Dr. Garell has served as president of the Society for Adolescent Medicine, chairman of the youth committee of the American Academy of Pediatrics, and as a forum member of the White House Conference on Children (1970) and White House Conference on Youth (1971). He has also been a member of the editorial board of the *American Journal of Diseases of Children*.

C. Everett Koop, M.D., Sc.D., is Surgeon General, Deputy Assistant Secretary for Health, and Director of the Office of International Health of the U.S. Public Health Service. A pediatric surgeon with an international reputation, he was previously surgeon-in-chief of Children's Hospital of Philadelphia and professor of pediatric surgery and pediatrics at the University of Pennsylvania. Dr. Koop is the author of more than 175 articles and books on the practice of medicine. He has served as surgery editor of the *Journal of Clinical Pediatrics* and editor-in-chief of the *Journal of Pediatric Surgery*. Dr. Koop has received nine honorary degrees and numerous other awards, including the Denis Brown Gold Medal of the British Association of Paediatric Surgeons, the William E. Ladd Gold Medal of the American Academy of Pediatrics, and the Copernicus Medal of the Surgical Society of Poland. He is a Chevalier of the French Legion of Honor and a member of the Royal College of Surgeons, London.